Dysfluencies

Dysfluencies

On Speech Disorders in Modern Literature

Chris Eagle

Bloomsbury Academic
An imprint of Bloomsbury Publishing Plc

B L O O M S B U R Y
NEW YORK • LONDON • NEW DELHI • SYDNEY

Bloomsbury Academic
An imprint of Bloomsbury Publishing Inc

1385 Broadway	50 Bedford Square
New York	London
NY 10018	WC1B 3DP
USA	UK

www.bloomsbury.com

BLOOMSBURY and the Diana logo are trademarks of Bloomsbury Publishing Plc

First published 2014
Paperback edition first published

Library of Congress Cataloging-in-Publication Data
A catalog record for this book is available from the Library of Congress.

ISBN: HB: 978-1-6235-6332-5
PB: 978-1-5013-0866-6
ePDF: 978-1-6235-6622-7
ePUB: 978-1-6235-6462-9

Typeset by Deanta Global Publishing Services, Chennai, India

For my teachers,
Kevin Miles
&
Maryann Black

Contents

Acknowledgments

During the research and writing of this book, I was repeatedly asked the same question by friends, colleagues, and strangers alike, whenever I shared my work with them. The question was what had drawn me to this "stuttering business" in the first place. My answer, I often noticed, would then be scrutinized for the minutest trace of a dysfluency in my speech, some stutter overcome, some hint of a lisp. The assumption, which many even made explicit, was that there had to be some personal motivation for me to write a book on such a "quirky" topic. As a matter of fact there was, but not the one most people suspected. The real motivation behind this book is the admiration I feel for how bravely (and comedically) my father handled his very difficult recovery from stroke and aphasia. Over the several months it took for his speech to return, a kind of private language developed between us—made up of mumbled code words and hand gestures—which I like to think has given me a much richer sense of what it means to communicate. So it is my father, first and foremost, whom I have to thank for this book. His uniquely "expressive aphasia" has inspired and informed every one of these pages.

My approach to medical history has been deeply influenced by three books that I would like to acknowledge here: L. S. Jacyna's *Lost Words*, Benson Bobrick's *Knotted Tongues*, and Howard Kushner's *A Cursing Brain*. The debt this book owes to theirs will be evident to any reader. I would also like to thank the aphasiologist Dr Hugh Buckingham for generously "diagnosing" several transcripts of modernist poetry for signs of jargonaphasia, as well as my dear friend Dr Ronald Workman for entertaining my many questions on clinical practice over the years.

I began the initial research for this book years ago, as a side project during the writing of my dissertation, so I have many friends to thank for their insights ever since the early stages of this project including Anna de Biasio, Mark Allison, Matt Losada, Matt Ritchie, Greg Fiorini, Shane Lillis, Dirk Van Hulle, Michael Jonik, Michael O'Sullivan, and the outstanding students of the seminar I taught on non-standard language at U. C. Berkeley. For their professional and personal guidance over the years, I would also like to express my gratitude to Professors Jan Rigaud, Michael Berthold, Walter Brogan, C. D. Blanton, Dorothy Hale, and Kevis Goodman. This book would not have been possible without the additional institutional support extended to me by Cindy Weinstein at Caltech and by Anthony Uhlmann at the Writing and Society Research Centre of the University of Western Sydney. While at U. W. S., my ideas have been tested and strengthened by my generous colleagues Chris Fleming, Lorraine Sim, and Chris Peterson.

Thanks of course go to my editor Haaris Naqvi for his thoughtful suggestions throughout the editorial process, and to my research assistant Lou Jillett for her painstaking correction of the final manuscript. Shorter versions of Chapters 3 and 4 were both previously published, in *Comparative Literature Studies* and *Philip Roth Studies*, respectively.

Finally and above all, I would like to thank Adeline Tran for her thoughtful responses to virtually every draft of every chapter. Without her steady encouragement and support, this project would have been started many times but certainly never finished.

Introduction: The Neurolinguistic Turn

"Dear Sir, It hath pleased almighty God this morning to deprive me of the powers of speech"

– Samuel Johnson (1783)

"Dear Mother, Since you insist I respond right away, you need to understand that writing my whole name is now a great task for my brain."

– Charles Baudelaire (1866)

On a June night in 1783, Samuel Johnson suffered a mild stroke in his London home which left the 73-year-old lexicographer unable to speak for several days. What we know of Doctor Johnson's cerebral vascular accident comes primarily from his autopathographic account in detailed letters he wrote to his friends and numerous doctors during the fortnight it took for his speech to return to normal. Overweight and suffering from increasingly poor health, Johnson was being treated at the time for a variety of conditions, including an asthmatic constriction of the chest, chronic insomnia, gouty legs and ankles, toothache, abdominal pains, and a painful swelling of one of his testicles.[1] On the afternoon prior to his stroke, Johnson had sat for his portrait at the studio of Miss Frances Reynolds. Afterward, he reports having walked a considerable distance, then going to bed at his regular hour, all without incident.

In the middle of the night, he was roused suddenly from his sleep, something which happened often due to the insomnia which he was treating with small doses of opium. On that particular night though, immediately upon waking, Johnson felt, in his words, "a confusion and indistinctness in my head."[2] Long fearful of the loss of his sanity, he devised an unusual method for testing his mental faculties. In what one neurologist has since called "the first aphasia testing," Johnson set himself the task of composing a short prayer in Latin, a quatrain imploring the Lord that, whatever should happen to his body, at least his reason should be spared.[3] To his relief, the writing of the verse came easily, and though he judged the short poem to be mediocre, the fact that he could judge its literary merits at all reassured him that his faculties remained intact for the time being.

The exact order of events that followed is not entirely clear from his account, but we know that soon after composing the verse, Johnson determined that he had suffered a "paralytic stroke" and the ability to speak had been taken from him. What seems most likely is that having composed the verse in his head, Johnson attempted to recite it aloud and, finding he could not, decided he was suffering not from madness but from paralysis. His first recourse was to break his vow of abstinence by drinking down two drams of brandy, "in order to rouse the vocal organs," as he put it, but rather than restoring his eloquence, the brandy only made him drift back to sleep.[4] In the morning, still unable to speak but able to write with slight difficulties, Johnson penned the following letter to his neighbor:

> Dear Sir,
> It hath pleased almighty God this morning to deprive me of the powers of speech; and, as I do not know but that it may be his farther good pleasure to deprive me soon of my senses, I request you will, on the receipt of this note, come to me, and act for me, as the exigencies of my case may require.
> I am, Sincerely Yours, S. Johnson. June 17th 1783.[5]

Several decades later, in the Spring of 1866, another man of letters, Charles Baudelaire, would suffer a stroke that was more severe and debilitating than the brief aphasic episode from which Doctor Johnson recovered in a matter of weeks. In 1864, Baudelaire had relocated to Brussels to escape his Parisian creditors and to seek out an interested publisher for his collected works. While living in Brussels, he was beset with "various minor infirmities, rhumatisms, and neuralgias, etc." which he described in letters to his mother, Madame Aupick, under the title of his "Belgian Health."[6] The ill effects of the Belgian climate on the 45-year-old *poète maudit* left him bedridden sometimes for days on end with chronic diarrhea and heart palpitations. Just 2 months before his stroke, Baudelaire finally decided to heed the advice of his friends and return to France.

Before ending his stay in Belgium, Baudelaire wished to revisit his favorite Baroque church, the Eglise de Saint-Loup in the town of Namur, which he had written about in his recent book *Pauvre Belgique*. On 15 March 1866, he took the train from Brussels to tour the church with two of his friends, the illustrator Félicien Rops and his publisher Auguste Poulet-Malassis. As Baudelaire stood admiring one of the church's ornate confessionals, he collapsed onto the marble floor. In the days that followed, Baudelaire's behavior as well as his speech patterns would show increasing signs of confusion. On the train ride back to Brussels, he asked his friends to open (rather than close) an already open window. A few days later, after an evening out with another friend, the photographer Neyt, Baudelaire said "see you tonight" (rather than "goodbye") as they parted.[7] Concerned over his friend's speech blunders and strange demeanor, Neyt went back to check on Baudelaire that same night. He eventually found him alone and particularly unwell in a local tavern. With some difficulty, Neyt managed to help Baudelaire back to his room. When he returned to look in on him again in the morning, he found Baudelaire fully dressed in bed. According to Neyt, the poet's eyes opened, "but he remained perfectly still and was unable to say a word."[8]

The initial diagnosis was meningitis of the left hemisphere, with resulting hemiplegia of the right side and subsequent aphasia. When his condition worsened, the decision was made to hospitalize Baudelaire at the Institut Saint-Jean et Sainte-Elisabeth in Brussels, where on 26 March his aphasia briefly subsided enough for him to dictate a letter to his doctor in which he indicated to his mother the current state of his language:

> Dear Mother, Since you insist I respond right away, you need to understand that writing my whole name now is a great task for my brain.
> – Charles Baudelaire, 1866
>
> [Ma chere mère, Puisque tu éxige que je te réponde de suite, il faut que tu sache que écrire mon nom de travers est un grand travail de cerveau pour moi. – Charles, March 26th, 1866][9]

Read alongside each other, these two letters by Johnson and Baudelaire perfectly illustrate the major paradigm shift which takes place in the decades between their two strokes: from the traditional conception of language as a spiritual faculty to the modern view of language as a biological process rooted in the brain. More importantly, their remarks on their respective *losses* of language also serve to illustrate the central topic of this book, namely, the new ways in which disorders of speech and language are understood (and in some cases experienced firsthand) by modern writers, and how these varied forms of language breakdown are in turn represented in modern literature.

Occurring when they do, the two strokes of Doctor Johnson and Baudelaire can also be said to bookend the emergence of modern neurolinguistics, beginning with the much-maligned attempts by the phrenologist Franz Gall (starting in 1798) to localize our higher faculties in specific regions of the brain and culminating several decades later with the landmark case studies of Paul Broca (1861–67), which more definitively established the left hemisphere of the brain as the "site" [siège] of articulated language. Completed in August 1861, Broca's "Notes on the site of the faculty of articulated language, followed by an observation of aphemia" offers a comprehensive pathographical account of a French farmer named Leborgne, who was transferred to Broca's surgical ward at Bicêtre Hospital on 11 April 1861.[10] Born in 1810, Leborgne had suffered epileptic attacks from an early age, but he was able to continue farming until the onset of his aphasia at the age of 30. It is not known whether Leborgne lost the ability to speak gradually or suddenly, but when he was first admitted as a patient at Bicêtre, he had been speechless for approximately 3 months. Only one monosyllable remained available to him, the nonsense word "*tan*," which he would repeat twice in quick succession ("*tan tan*") in response to any question posed to him. Monsieur Tan, as he soon came to be known, would spend the remaining 21 years of his life at Bicêtre, never recovering the ability to speak. He spent his first 10 years on the ward in otherwise perfect health. Then, at the age of 40, the muscles in his right arm gradually fell into complete paralysis. This paralysis quickly spread through his right leg until he was unable to walk. When he was finally transferred to the care of Dr Broca, Tan had been bedridden and speechless for 7 full years. He died only 6 days later, and Broca performed the autopsy on his brain within 24 hours of his death.

The conclusions Broca would draw from this case regarding the cerebral localization of language attained a degree of irrefutablity never achieved by Broca's predecessors, thanks to the rare opportunity to combine a detailed medical history of the patient together with a firsthand clinical examination and postmortem of the patient's brain. Before Tan's death on 17 April, Broca subjected him to an extensive series of neurological and physiological tests in order to eliminate other possible contributing factors to his language loss. Broca found that Tan's only significant impairment in the final week of his life, beyond the aphasia itself, was the progressive paralysis of his right side. The proper functioning of Tan's nervous system was confirmed by his "flinching and screams" at certain incisions Broca made.[11] Although Tan had difficulty swallowing (dysphagia), the organs of speech functioned normally. "The tongue was not at all paralyzed," notes Broca, and "the muscles of the larnyx did not seem impaired at all, the timbre of the voice was natural, and the sounds the patient made in pronouncing his monosyllable were perfectly pure."[12] In tests of the patient's intelligence, Broca was also able to confirm that Tan was at least "more intelligent than is required for speaking."[13] Tan understood most if not all questions put to him. He knew his own age as well as the number of years he had spent at the hospital, which he could verify with gestures from his unparalyzed left hand. When Broca asked him to describe the progression of his disease, Tan pointed first to his tongue, then to his arm and leg. Prior to conducting the autopsy, Broca was therefore highly confident that he had narrowed the cause of Tan's language loss down to a single determining factor, which he predicted would be a lesion somewhere in the frontal lobe of the left hemisphere. Broca did find substantial damage from lesions to the second and third convolutions of the left frontal lobe, confirming his hypothesis. Based upon these findings, Broca made the epochal declaration during his presentation of Tan's brain to his fellow members of the Society of Anthropology: "All evidence leads us to believe in this case that the lesion to the frontal lobe was the cause of the loss of speech."[14]

In the full report published 4 months later in the *Bulletins de la Société Anatomique*, Broca begins by crediting his precursor Jean-Baptiste Bouillaud with salvaging the theory of cerebral localization from what he calls "the shipwreck of phrenology." This is not to suggest that Broca was wholly critical of the phrenological school. On the contrary, he credits Franz Gall as the first to "place the site of the language faculty in the frontal part of the brain."[15] But Bouillaud, in his estimation, had made two crucial modifications to Gall's original hypothesis, modifications which Broca saw as the true foundation of his own work. The first was to avoid considering language as a simple faculty depending on a single cerebral organ. The second was to expand the size of the area thought to control language beyond the couple of millimeters Gall had accorded to it. In Bouillaud's 1825 *Recherches Cliniques*, as well as in numerous later studies, Broca's predecessor had broadened the size of what he termed the "legislative center of language" to include the entire left frontal lobe.[16] Decades before Broca, Bouillaud also asserted that language loss was linked definitively to lesions in this relatively broad area. With the case of Tan, Broca struck a balance between what he saw as the overcircumscribed position of Gall and the undercircumscribed position of Bouillaud, by shifting the focus to "the convolutions that the phrenologists made the great mistake of neglecting."[17] The new modern field of aphasiology, as Broca construed it, was at its roots therefore still phrenological, but it was now "the phrenology of convolutions and not the phrenology of bumps."[18]

The second case study of language loss that Broca would conduct later that same year has received much less attention in aphasia studies, yet it was in many ways more important for the theory of cerebral localization than the celebrated case of Tan. Published in November 1861, Broca's "New observation of aphemia produced by a lesion in the posterior half of the second and third frontal convolutions" would provide him with that crucial second case needed to reconfirm his previous findings.[19] This second aphemic patient was an 84-year-old man named Lelong, who was admitted to Bicêtre on 27 October 1861 and died a short 2 weeks later. Following an apoplectic attack in the Spring of 1860, Lelong's vocabulary had been permanently reduced to five simple words: *oui, non, trois, toujours,* and a truncated form of his own name, *Lelo.* Broca was again able to eliminate other contributing factors such as diminished intelligence or paralysis of the speech organs prior to the patient's death. Upon autopsy, he found that "in comparing the two brains [those of Monseiur Tan and Lelong] we can establish the center of the lesion as *identically the same* in the two cases."[20] Due to the much shorter span between the onset of Lelong's aphasia and his death (only 18 months), Lelong's brain provided even stronger evidence of the link between lesions to the second and third convolutions and language loss. Lelong's lesion was "incomparably more circumscribed than that which existed in the brain of Tan," and there was none of the degeneration of brain matter that had complicated diagnosis in the previous case.[21] All of these facts emboldened Broca to declare it incontestable that damage to the two convolutions had been "the direct cause of the aphemia."[22] From this point, the inference from localization of symptom to localization of function was much easier to make. Since the integrity of the third frontal convolution of the left hemisphere (still known today as "Broca's area") was essential to the production of speech, this area had to be the very site of articulated language.

In order to clarify the specific nature of the pathology he had uncovered, Broca distinguished three different levels (espèces) of language, each of which can be subject to different impairments. At the highest level, our "general language faculty" is defined as "the faculty of establishing a constant relationship between an idea and a sign."[23] This general faculty encompasses virtually all forms of signification, including "speech, mime, typing, picture writing, phonetic writing, etc."[24] The second level includes all the various faculties responsible for converting our ideas into signs, whether those signs are gestural, written, or articulated as speech. Lastly, the third and most basic level contains the complex set of muscular and neural operations needed to produce meaningful messages, again whether through gesture, writing, or voice. With Tan, whose actual verbal production was almost nil, Broca was careful to point out that the man's impairment was nonetheless restricted to a single faculty within the second level of language:

> This loss of speech in individuals who are neither paralyzed nor idiots constitutes a very specific symptom for which I consider it useful to invent a special name. So I will name it aphemia (alpha-privative, *phemi* = I speak, I pronounce); for it is only the faculty of articulating words that these patients lack. They hear and understand everything that is said to them; they are in full possession of their senses; they produce vocal sounds without difficulty; they execute with their tongue and lips movements that are far more elaborate and energetic than is required for the articulation of sounds; and yet the perfectly sensible answer that they would like to give is reduced to a very small number of articulated sounds, always the same ones and always arranged in the same way; their vocabulary, if one may call it that, consists of a short series of syllables, sometimes of one monosyllable expressing everything or rather expressing nothing, for this single word is most of the

time unknown to any existing vocabulary. For some patients not even this
bit of articulated language is left; in vain they struggle without pronouncing
a single syllable.[25]

It is apparent from this first definition of his new pathology that Broca was
determined to differentiate the aphemic patient's symptoms from outwardly
similar symptoms with which it had been too often confused historically, such
as idiocy or deaf-mutism. Elsewhere, Broca would justify the need to coin an
entirely new term on philological grounds. In an 1864 letter to his colleague
Armand Trousseau, he argued that available terms like "aphonia" and "alalia"
would only prolong these confusions due to their classical associations (dating
back to Galen and Hippocrates) with the loss of voice and deaf-mutism,
respectively.[26] Above all, however, Broca was intent on separating aphemia
from paralysis of the speech organs. He points out, for instance, how Tan
himself mistakenly "attributed his loss of speech to paralysis of the tongue,
which was only natural."[27] So too in the case of Lelong, we are told that long
after his recovery from bodily paralysis, Lelong's daughter remained convinced
that her father's speechlessness was due to a "paralyzed tongue."[28] In other
words, the most likely diagnosis to a well-educated man like Samuel Johnson
had, by 1861, acquired the status of a folk-etiology which science must work
to overcome.

Needless to say, traces of this neurolinguistic turn hardly could have been
present as early as 1783 in the autopathography of Samuel Johnson. For the
devout Anglican, the human faculty of articulate speech belonged to God,
both to give and to take away. In letter after letter throughout his illness,
he reiterated that, "it has pleased God by a paralytic stroke in the night to
deprive me of speech," and that it was his humble hope that God "will spare
my understanding, and restore my speech."[29] From Boswell, we also know that
not 2 months before his stroke, in April 1783, Johnson affirmed his position
on the popular debate in his era over whether language was of human or
divine origin. Language, argues Johnson in Boswell's paraphrase, "must have
come by inspiration. A thousand, nay, a million of children could not invent a
language. While the organs are pliable, there is not understanding enough to
form a language; by the time that there is understanding enough, the organs
are become stiff."[30] Beyond this implausibility of human understanding ever

coinciding with a pliable tongue, there is for him the added implausibility of speech even occurring to primitive man as a possibility. Without the aid of God, Johnson suggests we would have no better chance of discovering our own ability to speak "than cows or hogs would think of such a faculty."[31]

As a self-described dabbler in physic, Johnson was quick to propose various remedies for his condition from the very first day of his illness. He began rather dangerously by administering two drams of fortified wine, as he later explained, because "wine has been celebrated for the production of eloquence."[32] Confident that his situation was not beyond remedy, Johnson next proposed the use of an emetic, wondering "if a vomit vigorous and rough would not rouse the organs of speech to action."[33] When his primary physician, Doctor Heberden, arrived, vesicatories were prescribed to blister his head and throat in an attempt to alleviate pressure on the organs of speech. It is a wonder how Johnson ever spoke again with a treatment regimen of drinking, vomiting, and blistering, but within a week he was in fact able to report to a friend, "my power of utterance improves daily."[34] What is of significance for our purposes here is that all of the prescribed remedies have in common the goal of restoring *language* by rousing the throat and tongue out of their paralysis. There is as yet nothing in Johnson's letters resembling the modern sense of language loss that comes in the wake of Broca, where the breakdown of the faculty of articulated language (so-called pure aphasia) is carefully distinguished from the motor paralysis of the tongue and the larnyx (apraxia or ataxia).[35] On the contrary, when Johnson finds himself able to utter the word *no*, but unable to utter the word *yes*, this peculiarity has nothing to do for him with a breakdown of word recall or the faculty of language as such. Rather, his inability to utter one word versus another is, Johnson assumes, simply because "my organs were so obstructed."[36] In other words, it is a matter of the tongue finding certain words more or less difficult to pronounce.

In the case of Baudelaire, there exists no detailed autopathography like that of Samuel Johnson to indicate his own sense of his aphasia, and so we must rely for the most part on secondhand accounts from his friends, his mother, and his doctors. It would seem, as several aphasiologists have concluded in posthumous case studies of the poet, that Baudelaire suffered not one but a series of strokes throughout March 1866, most likely hemorrhagic in nature and of increasing severity. The result was the virtually total loss of language sometimes referred to as global aphasia, with the related complications of alexia and agraphia leaving him equally unable to read or write.[37] By all accounts, for the next several months Baudelaire's speech was limited to one singularly unfortunate phrase, the blasphemous "*Cré Nom*" (short for "*Sacré Nom de Dieu*"), which he learned to pronounce with a variety of inflections to the horror of the Sisters of the Institut Saint-Jean, who pled with his mother to remove her son from their care.[38]

Curses are often the last words to go for many aphasics, but there is nonetheless quite a bit of irony in the fact that Samuel Johnson embraced the will of God in letter after letter, whereas Baudelaire literally seemed to his nurses to be cursing God for his fate. It could be said as well that there is an added poignancy to the aphasias of these particular men, the first great lexicographer of the English language and one of the greatest poets of the nineteenth century. Johnson, whose stated wish in the Preface to his great *Dictionary* was that words "might be less apt to decay and that signs might be permanent, like the things which they denote," suddenly found his own speech in a state of total decay, and Baudelaire, who was generally considered (much like Johnson) one of the great conversationalists of his age, was unable to write even a note without assistance or to recognize written words on the page, limited to a handful of words for expressing all of his wants and feelings.[39] Many of his friends reported Baudelaire's rage and desperation to make himself understood in the 2 weeks he spent at the Brussels clinic. When his bodily paralysis improved enough for him to walk with a cane, he was relocated to Paris. Until his death in the Fall of 1867, Baudelaire's verbal recovery was never more than slight. Months after his stroke, his vocabulary expanded to include five new words: *bonjour, bonsoir, monsieur, adieu*, and the name of his doctor. By November 1866, his improvements were still so slight that one finds his mother excitedly recounting that her son can now utter whole phrases such as "*la lune est belle*" and "*passez-moi la moutarde*."[40]

Although Baudelaire dictated only seven more letters after his initial attack on 15 March, and his correspondence ceases altogether after 30 March, the sole reference he does make to his language difficulties in the dictated letter of 26 March is still incredibly revealing as to how much thinking about language had changed by the mid-1860s. The "great task of the brain" [grand travail de cerveau] Baudelaire undergoes in writing his own name makes it patently clear that by 1866 an educated patient in his position would now grasp his language difficulties as an impairment of *the brain*.[41] In this respect, Baudelaire's simple comment to his mother marks the starting point of this study of the history of interactions between literary practice and speech pathology from 1861 to the present. Furthermore, the operative sense of "modern" literature for this study is primarily a clinical one, referring to works of literature written after 1861 (or post-Broca), that is, after the neurological view of both language and language loss begins to permeate the literary imagination.

During this timespan of roughly 150 years, I distinguish three distinct historical stages during which neurological and psychological views on language breakdown have competed for dominance, and my fundamental argument is that works of literature have responded differently to the issue of language breakdown as the dominant views on speech pathology have shifted: from neurological (1860s to 1920s) to psychological (1920s to 1980s), and back to neurological starting with the "decade of the Brain" (the 1990s to the present).

In order to demonstrate the direct impact of fields like neurology, aphasiology, psychopathology, and speech pathology as concretely as possible, I delve into the scientific and medical backgrounds of the various writers in this study, assessing how informed (or in some cases, misinformed) they are about the medical ideas of their times on the conditions they are representing. Building on this historiographic work, a second overarching claim I make in this book is that even those writers whose portrayals are extremely well informed by medical knowledge (e.g. Proust) still utilize speech disorders primarily as metaphors. Virtually without exception in modern literature, speech pathologies are "diagnosed" metaphorically as the symptom of some character flaw such as excessive nervousness or weakness, or treated as a symbol for the general tendency of language toward communicative breakdown, ambiguity, polysemy, misunderstanding, etc. Each of the chapters in this book will therefore address two basic questions: (1) the extent to which the portrayal of disordered speech accords with the medical knowledge of the time and (2) the metaphorical significance of the speech disorder beyond its clinical representation. While the works are studied for the most part in chronological order, because of the overarching historical argument this book makes, some of the chapters do connect works from different periods based on the metaphorical approach they share in common.

In Chapter 1, I begin by contextualizing the impact of nascent fields like neurology, physiology, and aphasiology on Zola's early development of his naturalist method in the late 1860s. From there, I address two related issues: first, the awareness Zola actually possessed of the new field of aphasiology while composing his first major novel *Thérèse Raquin* (1867), and second, how much that awareness does (or does not) inform his portrayal of language loss in the case of the character Madame Raquin, who, late in the novel, loses her ability to speak following a stroke. Her language loss, I argue, is portrayed not as an impairment of the brain (in line with Broca's discoveries), but in more traditional pre-Broca terms (not unlike those expressed by Samuel Johnson) as a paralytic impairment of her tongue and throat. In terms of Zola's place in the history of portrayals of speech pathology, this chapter argues therefore that *Thérèse Raquin* stands in a more transitional moment, one where the discourse of neurology is already prevalent but that of aphasiology has not yet been fully carried over into literature. Aphasia and paralysis are subjects that Zola revisits throughout his career, and as I show, it is not until *La Terre* (1887) that Zola's depiction of language loss truly approaches a post-Broca understanding of the aphasic condition as a neurogenic impairment of the language faculty as such. In the second half of Chapter 1, I go on to show how the discourse of aphasiology was further assimilated into the modern novel through Marcel Proust's interactions with leading members of the neurological and aphasiological communities of Paris. Beginning in the 1870s and 1880s, one of the major debates among aphasiologists was over whether the aphasic's difficulty in producing words was due to an impairment of the language faculty or an impairment of memory. Many believed that aphasia was ultimately a form of word-amnesia, a forgetting of words rather than a breakdown of language. What is not well known is that one of the major figures in this debate was Marcel Proust's father Adrien Proust, who published two important monographs on aphasia in the 1870s. Biographers of Marcel Proust have also noted his crippling fear that he would develop aphasia himself, following his mother's stroke. Building on this historical and biographical context, I demonstrate the central importance of neurological and psychopathological views of language breakdown to Proust's project. Language throughout the *Recherche* is rendered as an ultimately fragile medium, susceptible to breakdown through parapraxes, malapropisms, and what are known as paraphasias, the temporary forgetting of words to which we are all prone. Focusing on the "case study" of the Baron de Charlus, who regresses in the *Recherche* from the novel's greatest raconteur to an aphasic who must struggle, in the final volume, to produce a single word, I argue that Proust's portrayal of Charlus exemplifies the tension in the early twentieth century between neurogenic and psychogenic accounts of language breakdown.

In Chapter 2, I show how the sense of language as an ultimately fragile medium developed by Proust reaches its peak during World War I, as thousands of new cases of head wounds and shell shock increase public awareness of conditions like aphasia as well as the phenomena of war stammering and war mutism. Drawing on L. S. Jacyna's writings on the history of aphasiology and Peter Leese's definitive study of war neurosis *Shell Shock*, I begin this chapter by elaborating the competing theories (neurogenic vs. psychogenic) during the War about the etiologies of various speech disorders brought on by trench warfare. From there, the chapter focuses on the case of the World War I poet Wilfred Owen, who was admitted to Craiglockhart War Hospital in 1917 for shell shock and experienced war stammering firsthand. My analysis of Owen's poetry focuses on the tensions between voice, silence, and noise which he creates in his war poems, primarily through his distinctive use of onomatopoeia. I also reflect on how his personal experience with war stammering fostered those tensions and informed his conception of the most authentic poetic response to the traumas of war.

Chapter 3 completes the shift to the second historical phase, where psychogenic accounts of language breakdown take precedence over neurogenic ones, due to the emergence of Freudianism in the 1920s. Beginning with Virginia Woolf's portrait of the stammerer Septimus Smith, I demonstrate how the commonplace association during World War I between soldiering and stuttering gradually transforms into a popular psychogenic conception of the personality type of the stutterer as neurotic, timid, and sexually repressed.

Taking Melville's Billy Budd as an archetype for virtually all portrayals of the stuttering male that follow, I argue that the portrayals of the stuttering young man by Ken Kesey and Yukio Mishima share a tendency to understand the stutter in two interrelated ways: to diagnose it in oedipal terms as a form of psychosexual "blockage" in which sexual inexperience causes stuttered speech and to diagnose the stutter metaphorically as the symptom of an underlying character flaw symbolic of the postwar male.

In Chapter 4, I take up the ways in which stuttering and mutism have been metaphorized in relation to issues of violence and political voice in novels by Robert Graves, Philip Roth, and the Australian novelist Gail Jones. The eponymous narrator of Graves' historical novel *I, Claudius* (1934) bears obvious affinities to King George VI, another reluctant stammering monarch, who took the throne in 1936. With this political backdrop in mind, I show how the stutter acts in Graves' novel as a symbol for Claudius' struggle to balance the violence of monarchical power with his goal of restoring "free speech" by making Rome a republic again. From there, I turn to two contemporary portrayals of young women who stutter in Philip Roth's *American Pastoral* (1998) and Gail Jones' *Sorry* (2007). Statistically speaking, stuttering is significantly less common in women than in men, and its portrayal with women in fiction is even rarer. The portrayals of stuttering in the female characters Merry Levov and Perdita Keene, nevertheless, share the extremely common conception, dating back to *Billy Budd*, of the stutterer as prone to violent, destructive behavior. I argue that Roth and Jones deploy the stutter not only in gendered terms, as a symbol of the suppression of the female voice, but also in broader terms, as a symbol of the way that struggles to achieve political voice in the face of injustice often result in violence.

Finally, Chapter 5 marks the return of neurogenic views to literature, coinciding with the resurgence of interest in brain research in the 1990s. The most interesting example of this new neurally inflected literature is Jonathan Lethem's recent portrayal of Tourette's syndrome in *Motherless Brooklyn* (1999) in which the narrator Lionel Essrog understands his condition in explicitly neurological terms as a disease of the brain. The involuntary verbal tics and copralalic outbursts common to sufferers of Tourette's syndrome represent a very different model of language breakdown from those treated in Chapters 1–4, in that tourettic speech is not an inability or difficulty with producing words, but rather an inability to restrain the production of words. In Lionel's case, I show how his lack of control over the language that flows out of him is understood deterministically as a neurological condition. In this respect, Lethem's neurophysiological approach to his narrator-protagonist represents a kind of neo-naturalism, situating *Motherless Brooklyn* in the same tradition as Zola's *Thérèse Raquin*. What separates Lethem's naturalism from Zola's, however, is that Lionel is fully conscious (unlike Zola's characters) of his own neural determinism (overinformed as it were for a patient) and consequently able to measure the exact extent to which his tourettic speech is within or beyond his control. The result is a distinctly postmodern approach not only to disordered speech, but also to the dividing line between public and private selves. Of course, this latter issue underlies all the chapters of this book as well. If speech is our most immediate instrument for giving account of ourselves to others, then disorderly speech in all of these texts conveys a sense of disjuncture between an individual's interiority and their public self that is endemic to modern life.

Aphasia and Neurology in Zola and Proust

"There is no case on record – at all events, I have never come across it – of a hero or heroine in a novel possessing a disagreeable voice."
                                          – Arthur Lovell, *Beauty of Tone in Speech and Song* (1904)

"la vieille paralytique"

In his 1889 monograph *De L'aphasie et de ses diverses formes*, the professor of medicine Désiré Bernard singled out Emile Zola as the sole example to date of a writer of fiction who had portrayed the condition of aphasia with any degree of clinical accuracy: "If a place ought to be reserved in this study for Letters, one would have to mention above all M. Emile Zola who, as early as 1867, portrayed an aphasic in the moving pages of *Thérèse Raquin*, with a perfect understanding of what he was describing."[1] This favorable assessment of the depiction of language loss in the story of Madame Raquin raises familiar questions about the more general role that scientific and medical discourses play throughout Zola's corpus. In terms of this study, Bernard's remark raises two other more specific questions: first, about the awareness Zola would have actually possessed of aphasiology during the year he spent composing his first major novel and second, whether the character Madame Raquin can in fact be properly termed "aphasic." To address these questions, I will examine two portrayals of language loss by Zola, the case of Madame Raquin and a second case of apoplexy and language loss from Zola's 1886 novel *La Terre*.

Désiré Bernard's passing reference to Zola comes in a footnote to the second chapter of *De L'aphasie*, in which he offers the polemical overview of aphasiology for which his study is remembered if at all today. Bernard's polemical ire is directed at those revisionist medical writers such as the

American neurologist William Hammond who, in the wake of Broca, had gone searching throughout Western history for prior evidence of aphasia being mentioned across the disciplines, in the works of philosophers like Plato and Sextus Empiricus, historians like Thucydides, grammarians like Suetonius, poets like Homer and Goethe, even the prophet Isaiah.[2] While Bernard does not deny that, "there have been aphasics as long as man has spoken and his brain has been prone to disease," he insists at the same time that any talk of aphasia *per se* prior to Broca's 1861 discovery was absurd since before then, "a total obscurity reigned over the alterations of language, as much in the clinical descriptions as in the nosologies."[3] In other words, for Bernard along with many of his contemporaries, aphasia as such simply did not exist until the discovery that lesions to the third frontal convolution of the left hemisphere consistently resulted in diverse forms of language loss. For the same reason, the Aphasic, either as a clinical or social category, could not exist yet either. In his historical study of aphasiology *Lost Words*, L. S. Jacyna notes the following in reference to Bernard's remarks on Zola: "It was only after Broca had described the condition that it became possible for aphasia to possess a textual existence. If one were to seek a true account of the condition in imaginative literature, it was necessary to look to writing in the modern, post-1861 period."[4] From this vantage point, Bernard's crediting of Zola with the first accurate literary portrayal of aphasia takes on a much greater significance, one in which the character of Madame Raquin could even be said to signal a new period in the history of the Novel where the neurological conception of language crossed for the very first time over into literature. If this were true, if Madame Raquin could be called "literature's first Aphasic," this would require of course that the textual existence of Zola's "old paralyzed woman" [vieille paralytique] be fully informed by a post-1861 view of the cerebral site of language as well as the cerebral cause of language loss.[5] But for reasons that will become clear over the course of this chapter, the depiction of Madame Raquin's paralysis and language loss does not ultimately bear this out, and it is not until slightly later, in 1886, that we find Zola depicting language loss in a distinctly post-Broca way.

What makes Bernard and Jacyna's assumption problematic from the start is the total absence of any biographical evidence that Zola, prior to composing

Thérèse Raquin, was familiar with Broca's case studies or with their reception in the medical circles of 1860s Paris. In his correspondence, Zola makes no mention of Broca or of his phrenological precursors Gall and Bouillaud. Nor is there any evidence in the years following, as Zola progresses through the *Rougon-Macquart* series, of a familiarity with the second wave of aphasiologists like Carl Wernicke, Adrien Proust (whose influence on his son I will discuss later in this chapter), *et al.* Although Zola does make occasional references in his letters to the work of Jean-Martin Charcot, Charcot's studies of aphasia were not conducted until long after the completion of *Thérèse Raquin* (circa 1883–84).[6] In the "case" of Madame Raquin, the symptoms that Désiré Bernard calls aphasic are nowhere in the novel referred to in those terms. Rather, the onset of Madame's health troubles is described more in line with the autopathography of Samuel Johnson, as a slowly progressive paralysis that first diminishes mobility in her lower limbs and gradually works its way upward to the vocal organs:

> Little by little paralysis was coming over Madame Raquin, and they foresaw the day when she would be chair ridden, powerless in body and mind. The poor old soul was beginning to mutter disconnected phrases, her voice was failing, and her limbs one after another were becoming useless.[7]

Madame is consistently referred to thereafter as "the paralyzed woman" [la paralytique], and her eventual language loss several months after the onset of her bodily paralysis is treated as the culmination of this immobility in the speech organs:

> Paralysis, which for months past had been creeping through her limbs, ever on the point of striking, seized her by the throat and pinioned her body. One evening, as she was quietly talking to Thérèse and Laurent, she stopped in the middle of a sentence, open-mouthed, gaping, feeling as if she were being strangled. She tried to shout for help but could only utter raucous sounds. Her tongue had turned to stone. Her hands and feet had stiffened. She was struck dumb and motionless [Elle se trouvait frappée de mutisme et d'immobilité].[8]

Although the term "aphasic" appears nowhere in the novel, we see here that Madame Raquin's loss of speech is explicitly referred to as a case of mutism.

Traditionally, mutism has been associated with either diminished intelligence (idiocy) or deafness. As we noted in the Introduction, Broca's main objective in coining the term "aphemia" was to differentiate the cerebral impairment of the language faculty from conditions with which they were confused, in particular, mutism and paralysis of the speech organs. In Zola's descriptions of Madame Raquin, however, her language loss is directly associated with both of these conditions. Her lips are described in paralytic terms as "twisted and inert" [tordues et inertes].[9] Likewise, her tongue has "turned to stone" [devenue de pierre], feels "cold against her palate" [froide contre son palais], and in the end falls "quite dead" [bien morte].[10] In terms of the dichotomy established in the Introduction, then, her language difficulties are clearly a matter of the tongue and throat, not of the brain. What is portrayed here is a breakdown of *speech*, not of the language faculty as such, something which contradicts Désiré Bernard's "diagnosis" of Madame Raquin as the first aphasic character in modern fiction.[11] This is not meant to argue of course that Madame does or does not suffer from aphasia, but simply that Zola's emphasis on paralysis and mutism means her language loss is still being portrayed (and most likely understood) in a pre-Broca sense. In terms of its place in the history of portrayals of speech pathology, *Thérèse Raquin* therefore stands in a more transitional moment, one where the discourse of neurology is already prevalent but that of aphasiology has not yet been fully assimilated into popular discourse.

"nervous being"

While there may be no direct evidence that Zola was familiar with the most current aphasiological theories at the time, the more general influence of mid-nineteenth-century positivism and biological science on Zola's early writings has been well documented.[12] It has also been more firmly established that the theory of heredity in Doctor Prosper Lucas' *Traité philosophique et physiologique de l'hérédité naturelle* (1850) and, most importantly, the methods of experimental physiology in Claude Bernard's *Introduction à l'étude de la médicine expérimentale* (1865) both had a direct impact on the radically new novelistic method that Zola developed for *Thérèse Raquin*. In his Preface to the second edition of the novel, Zola mixes various medical and scientific discourses to explicate his new method. His stated aim is to banish the customary psychological categories of character, motivation, personality, etc. around which the Novel was traditionally organized. Instead, he claims to perform the strictest study possible of "temperaments and not characters" with equal attention paid to the role of heredity and environment in modifying what he refers to as the human organism.[13]

Above all, in his Preface, Zola borrows liberally from the discourses of neurology and physiology, stressing that he has chosen to study these particular organisms because his protagonists, Thérèse and Laurent, are "completely dominated by their nerves and blood," respectively.[14] In his Introduction to the novel, Hénri Mitterand points out that terms like nerves, neurosis, and neurology were already in widespread use as early as 1845 due to a burgeoning interest in the pathology of the nervous system. The popularization from 1840 to 1870 of neurological and physiological terms in dictionaries like *Landais*, *Bescherelle*, and *Larousse* means, according to Mitterand, that "the link is very quickly established, in this domain, between the experts, the popularisers, the essayists, the critics and the novelists. . . . *Anatomy, scalpel, physiology, analysis, hysteria, neurosis, dissection, erethism*, are the buzzwords [maître-mots] of 1860."[15]

The popularization of the discourse of aphasia, on the other hand, happened much more gradually. The relatively slower assimilation of aphasiological terminology into popular discourse was due in part to the debates in the 1860s within the nascent field of aphasiology over which term best described this new pathology. Broca, as we know, considered a number of different terms (alogia, alalia, aphasia, aphemia, etc) to categorize the related forms of language loss his patients exhibited, however, the coinage he eventually chose (aphemia) was soon overtaken by Trousseau's preferred term (aphasia). In his 1864 letter to Trousseau, Broca objected to this because of a philosophical sense the word aphasia still carried in the 1860s, a sense which is now completely obsolete. The earliest known usage of "aphasia" was by the Stoic Sextus Empiricus, who used the word as a philosophical term to signify "a condition of mind, according to which we neither affirm nor deny anything."[16] This sense of aphasia as the antonym to phatic speech in propositional logic was anything but archaic by the

1860s. In fact, it persists as the primary definition in the *Larousse* dictionary of 1866 (the year before *Thérèse Raquin* was written), in which "aphasia" is defined as follows: "Indecision, one's state of mind in the case of questionable judgment" [Indécision, état de l'esprit dans le cas de jugement problématique].[17] It is not until the 1890 supplement of *Larousse* that the medical sense of aphasia as "loss of speech" [perte de la parole] supplants the philosophical sense and becomes the primary definition. Somewhat surprisingly, the 1863 dictionary of Broca's colleague Emile Littré also contains no entry for aphasia or aphemia, and it is not until the 1892 supplement of *Littré* that aphasia is finally defined in specific relation to the work of Broca as the "abolition of articulated language despite the faculty of expression remaining intact" [abolition du langage articulé malgré la persistence de la faculté d'expression].[18] Thus, to borrow Mitterand's formulation, terms like *aphasia* and *aphasic, aphemia* and *aphemic, alalia, aphonia, agraphia,* etc. simply did not have the same level of popular currency that the buzzwords of neurology did when Zola was writing *Thérèse Raquin.*

It comes as little surprise then that *Thérèse Raquin* is saturated not with the terms of aphasiology but with a more strictly neurological vocabulary of nerves and nervousness. The "nervous energy" [énergie nerveuse] that permeates Zola's novel comes mainly from his monotonous use of the keywords "nerves" and "nervous."[19] Nerves in *Thérèse Raquin* are variously described as rebellious, strained, terrified, stiffened, shattered, etc. They are said to stretch and give way, to threaten, dominate, and irritate the characters, and the three members of the novel's central love triangle are constantly searching for ways to calm or ease their strained nerves. Zola further expands this neurological texture of his novel by including different cognates of the root-word "nerve," making Thérèse and Laurent so "enervated" [s'énervait] by the horror of Camille's death that the "enervations of the crime" [énervements du crime] ultimately produce in them an "acute neurosis" [névrose aiguë].[20] The adjective "nervous" is applied over two-dozen times throughout the course of the novel to numerous mental, emotional, or physical states ranging from nervous joy to nervous anguish. Moreover, the twitchy bodily movements generated by their nervous existence include an assortment of nervous shivers, shakes, and contractions. Following the murder of Camille in Chapter 12, the remaining 20 chapters are almost entirely concerned with Laurent's and Thérèse's unsuccessful efforts to settle what Zola refers to as their "nervous being" [être nerveux].[21] The intended effect of this neural vocabulary, of course, was to take what the Novel had traditionally treated as higher mental and moral states (soul, passion, conscience, etc.) and reduce them to what Zola believed were at root purely physiological manifestations (nerves, blood, flesh, etc).

Many critics have pointed out that Zola's study of the temperaments of the principal characters in *Thérèse Raquin* adheres closely to the medieval theory of humors with its four types of temperaments (sanguine, melancholic, lymphatic, and bilious). Camille, whose "ill-health had impoverished his blood," rendering him sickly and weak as a child, exhibits a lymphatic disposition.[22] Thérèse is forced to grow up in the sterile environment of Camille's room and coddled by her aunt Madame Raquin as if she too were a sick child. She is even given the same medicines her cousin takes, but this "enforced invalidism" fails to weaken the "boiling" African blood which she inherits from her mother, a native beauty from Oran.[23] When she is later compelled to marry her cousin Camille, Thérèse displays an "external tranquility that concealed terrible bursts of passion," and her "boiling blood and taut nerves" are said to constitute a nervous temperament.[24] Lastly, Laurent comes from "genuine peasant stock" and his virile, "full-blooded" body is characteristic of a sanguine temperament.[25] In the narration of what is an otherwise conventionally melodramatic plotline—Thérèse's and Laurent's adulterous affair escalating to the murder of Camille and the eventual suicide of the murderers—Zola constantly reverts to physiological explanations couched in the vocabulary of nerves and blood since his project as articulated in the Preface was to achieve a novel where the characters are approached as biological organisms, nothing more than "human animals" with no free will and "a complete absence of soul."[26]

In order to emphasize this absence of either free will or soul in his two protagonists, Zola gradually merges them into a single, unified organism the more Laurent's sanguine temperament comes into contact with Thérèse's nervous one. On the journey back from Saint-Ouen immediately after the murder of Camille, the assimilation of their separate organisms is symbolized by a hand-clasp through which the blood seems to circulate between and unify their bodies: "It seemed to Laurent and Thérèse that their blood-stream passed from the one to the other by way of their united hands" [que le sang de l'un allait dans la poitrine de l'autre en passant par leurs poings unis].[27] Also in the planning of the murder, Zola reduces the couple to a single brain: "They dared not peer down into the depths of their being, to the depths of that fevered unrest, which filled their brain with a sort of thick acrid mist" [Eux-mêmes n'osaient regarder au fond de leur être, au fond de cette fièvre trouble qui emplissait leur cerveau d'une sorte de vapeur épaisse et âcre].[28] In addition to the singularizing of their shared brain (leur cerveau, rather than leurs cerveaux, which some translators have incorrectly translated as "brains"), it is significant that Zola does not refer to the couple's bond in their plan to murder Camille as a shared *esprit*, which would suggest a higher (psychological or spiritual) sense of mind or spirit. Instead, he chooses the more strictly anatomical term "cerveau" to indicate that their mental state, as well as their decision-making, is merely the product of a shared neurophysiology. The descriptions of their interactions increasingly reflect this sense of a biological process, of matter transferring back and forth, where Thérèse's nerves and Laurent's blood are said to mix together and establish a sort of equilibrium between their very different temperaments:

> Thérèse's highly-strung nature had acted in a strange way upon the stolid, sanguine one of Laurent. Formerly, when their passion was at its height, the differences between their temperaments had bound this man and this woman closely together, establishing a kind of balance between them in which each, as it were, completed the other's organism [en complétant pour ainsi dire leur organisme]. The lover contributed his blood and the mistress her nerves, they lived in each other, needing each other's embraces to regulate the mechanism of their being.[29]

Again, the singularity of their organism [leur organisme] reinforces this sense of the couple as a unified biological entity, a mechanism that is governed by biological laws and regulates itself through the mutual exchange of their blood and nerves.

Zola appears to have based his conception of the physiological interdependence of blood and nerves on the idea of the *circulus* developed by Claude Bernard in his *Introduction à l'étude de la médecine expérimentale*. In his 1880 essay *Le Roman expérimental*, Zola returns to Bernard in an attempt to integrate the principles of experimental physiology into the naturalist method. Insisting that the words doctor and novelist are virtually interchangeable, Zola argues that just as science seeks to explain the laws of the physical world, so too the novelistic project should entail the analysis of the laws of human behavior from a detached biological standpoint. What is surprising is that this late essay discusses Claude Bernard's theory of the *circulus* in detail without ever making any explicit reference back to *Thérèse Raquin*, even though Zola's treatment of the symbiotic temperaments of Thérèse and Laurent parallels Bernard's description of the *circulus vital* almost exactly:

> In complex organisms the organism of life actually forms a closed circle, but a circle which has a head and a tail in this sense, that vital phenomena are not all of equal importance, though each in succession completes the vital circle. Thus the muscular and nervous organs sustain the activity of the organs preparing the blood; but the blood in its turn nourishes the organs which produce it. Here it is an organic or social interdependence which sustains a sort of perpetual motion, until some disorder or stoppage of a necessary vital unit upsets the equilibrium, or leads to disturbance or stoppage in the play of the animal machine.[30]

In the same chapter where Bernard outlines this equilibrium established through the circulatory process of nerves and blood simultaneously sustaining each other, he also details the related possibility of a "dérangement organique" whereby one element in the circulus causes a breakdown of the entire system. Appropriating this idea in *Le Roman expérimental*, Zola argues that if the aim of the experimentalist doctor is to find the "simple initial cause" of this dislocation of the organism, then the experimental novelist should analogously locate the initial disturbance or blockage of the "social circulus." In the plot of *Thérèse Raquin*, the initial disturbance of Laurent's and Thérèse's equilibrium occurs when outside circumstances prevent the lovers from secretly meeting, thus pushing them to murder Camille, which then causes each of their temperaments to be thrown off balance:

> But something had gone out of gear. Thérèse's overwrought nerves had taken control, and suddenly Laurent had found himself thrown into a state of nervous hypersensitivity; under her sensual influence his own temperament had turned into that of a girl in a highly neurotic condition. It would be

interesting to study the modifications that sometimes take place in certain organisms as a result of predetermined circumstances. These modifications originate in the body but rapidly spread to the brain and thence to the whole individual.[31]

In this applied study of Bernard's notion of organic disarrangement, Thérèse experiences only an "undue stimulation of her normal nature," whereas Laurent's sanguine temperament acquires more and more of Thérèse's nerves until "the nervous side . . . took precedence over the sanguine, and this single fact modified his whole nature."[32] Thereafter, Laurent's organism suffers from regular attacks of nerves, described as "some fell disease, a sort of murder-hysteria, for the term disease or nervous disorder was really the only suitable one for Laurent's panics."[33] Out of this neurophysiological process of enervation comes a new social typology of modern urban life, what Zola calls the "new individual." This type emerges as Laurent's sanguine temperament grows more and more enervated by its contact with that of Thérèse: "This haggard, shuddering creature, the new individual who had just emerged from the lumping, oafish peasant, was now going through the fears and anxieties of nervous temperaments" [l'être frissonnant et hagard, le nouvel individu qui venait de se dégager en lui du paysan épais et abruti, éprouvait les peurs, les anxiétés des tempéraments nerveux].[34] The new individual, or nervous being, which Laurent comes to represent is a category that functions at once socially and medically, in that his enervation is physiologically triggered by his new urban environment. Although Laurent's speech is not directly impacted, as we will see in later chapters, he still serves as a kind of prototype for the many stutterers and ticcers of twentieth- and twenty-first-century literature, insofar as his nervous being is a mixture of neurophysiology and the environmental pressures of the modern city.

"raucous sounds"

Throughout his career, Zola returns again and again to these derangements of the brain. The result is that stroke, or apoplexy as it was known in the nineteenth century, is one of the more frequently occurring diseases across his corpus. Now outdated as a medical term, apoplexy derives from the Greek *apoplexia*, meaning to strike down, because the Greeks believed that the sudden loss of consciousness and paralysis came from being struck down by the Gods. In Zola's time, the term apoplexy encompassed any sudden loss of consciousness and subsequent paralysis, understood as being brought on by a rush of blood into an organ or tissue. Apoplexy was thus closely but not always exactly synonymous with our modern understanding of stroke as a cerebrovascular accident. For this reason, any illness that produced a sudden loss of consciousness could potentially be misdiagnosed as apoplexy.[35] In the novel Zola himself considered his masterpiece, *La Terre*, there are not one but several apoplectic attacks, two of which result in temporary language loss. Early in the novel, a gentleman from Cloyes is said to have spent 50000 francs to improve his property "only to be struck down with apoplexy before the paint was dry."[36] When Old Fouan suffers his apoplectic attack late in the novel, he "did not move his head and seemed turned to stone," and the doctor diagnoses him with a "mild attack of cerebral congestion."[37] The peasant woman La Frimat has also been the caretaker of a paralyzed husband for many years. Finally, there is the case of Mouche whom Jean Macquart finds one night "laid out by an apoplectic fit" [foudroyé par une attaque d'apoplexie].[38]

It is not until the case of Mouche that Zola's depictions of apoplexy and aphasia truly approach a neurogenic (or post-Broca) understanding. When Jean Macquart discovers old Mouche lying at the bottom of a cart, he drives the dying man home to his two daughters, Françoise and Lise. After Lise sees her father's "flushed face of which one side was contorted as if it had been pulled violently upward," she tearfully pleads, "Dad, say something, won't you? What's the matter, tell us. What in God's name is the matter? *It's your head, is it, and that's why you can't say anything?*" [C'est donc dans la tête, que tu ne peux seulement rien dire?] (emphasis added).[39] This simple question signals the actual shift to the kind of post-Broca understanding and portrayal of aphasia that cannot be truly located in *Thérèse Raquin*. If we recall the case of Broca's patient Lelong, we see that Mouche's daughter Lise understands her father's sudden speechlessness in a way that Lelong's daughter just a few years earlier could not, that is, as an impairment of the head rather than a malfunctioning tongue.

While this later case clearly exhibits a much stronger connection between language and brain, it is important to note that Zola's use of the word "head" in *La Terre* is not restricted solely to neurological processes. Immediately after Mouche's stroke, his daughters become so distraught that when Jean asks where their father should be taken, the two girls are said to have "lost their heads [la tête perdue] and could not decide."[40] In this case, the word "head" operates more metaphorically than clinically to represent the daughters' emotional distress and not their physiology. This dual treatment of the head as both a scientific term and a literary symbol recalls many of Zola's physiological explanations in *Thérèse Raquin* which, as Andrew Rothwell has persuasively argued, must be read on literal and metaphorical levels simultaneously.[41] Alluding to a lecture Zola gave on Balzac, where the word "heart" is said to stand "half-way between the physiological and mental domains," Rothwell notes that the terms "blood" and "nerves" similarly are "physical terms historically loaded with conventional behavioural and emotional connotations". The very same point could be made about the word "head" in *La Terre*, where the term functions both literally, as a physiological explanation of Mouche's speechlessness, and within the very same scene metaphorically, as a more psychological symbol for his daughters' emotional distress.

If Mouche can be said to offer a more accurate representation of an aphasic character than Madame Raquin from a clinical standpoint, as I noted earlier, this would seem to be because Zola is ultimately more interested in disclosing the physiology of Thérèse and Laurent's shared brain than he is in disclosing the impaired brain of Madame Raquin. Shortly after the onset of her paralysis, Madame's presence becomes entirely objectified and the reader's access to her thoughts is filtered almost exclusively through the point of view of Laurent's and Thérèse's shared brain. At first, the couple depend on Madame Raquin's conversation to divert their thoughts away from the horror of their crime, but once Madame loses her speech, they can only perceive her as an inanimate object. Their panic over Madame Raquin turning into a mere thing leads them to care for her not out of sympathy for her total paralysis but out of a sense of the nightmare that awaits them when they are left without the presence of her voice for a few hours a night to distract them from their neurologically inflected guilt over the murder of Camille. Madame's objectification is underscored by the proliferation of things she is likened to in her paralyzed, mute condition. In the evenings, Madame sits facing Laurent and Thérèse like a cadaver with a face resembling a death mask.[42] Forgetting that she is in the room, the couple are said to confuse her for another piece of furniture, and Thérèse even uses her as a sort of prayer-kneeler where she can confess her sins. Throughout the day, Madame sits in her armchair, according to the narrator, like a package, a thing, a bundle of laundry, a statue, a doll, among other household objects. As Jacyna writes, "Zola's account of aphasia thus concentrates on the devastating effects of the condition for the status of the self, both as an actor in the social world, and in her own subjective interiority."[43] Even when she is not treated like an object, she is still infantilized by those around her. Thérèse's caretaking of her aunt is compared to caring for an infant, and on their Thursday night soirées, Madame's guests address her as if "conversing rationally with a statue, as little girls do with their dolls" [raisonnablement à une statue, comme les petites filles parlent à leur poupée].[44] By portraying her as having reverted to a state of infancy, Zola is of course playing with the Latin sense of the word *infans* meaning "without speech," which in Roman society possessed legal ramifications we will revisit in Chapter 4.

Once deprived of language, Madame Raquin is described not only as thing-like and child-like, but her speechlessness is also said to reduce her to a state of animality. The mouth that paralysis has turned to stone becomes like "jaws" [mâchoires] that Therese can only open "as one opens those of an obstinate animal."[45] The strange counterpoint in the novel to Madame's mute animality is the imagined loquacity of the family cat François, who seems almost human to Laurent and capable of bearing witness to their crimes in a way that Madame cannot. Late in the novel, the cat's incessant miaowing torments Laurent until he "persuaded himself that, like Madame Raquin, the cat knew all about the crime and would denounce him if ever a day came when he could speak."[46] To prevent this from happening, Laurent throws the cat against the wall, and the wounded creature spends the rest of the night "miaowing raucously" [en poussant des miaulements rauques].[47] These raucous miaows directly echo the raucous sounds Madame is said to make following her stroke, and lest the reader miss this connection, Zola calls our attention to the "certain similarity between the angry beast and the paralysed woman."[48] The inclusion of this talking cat has baffled Zola scholars for the most part, but this is arguably because the significance of Madame's language loss for Zola's early conception of naturalism has not been fully appreciated. If this early version of naturalism was to be the rigorously scientific study of human animals that Zola asserted in his Preface, then the classical idea of language, as a higher faculty that elevates *homo loquens* above all other animals, also had to be discarded along with soul, conscience, free will, etc. From this vantage point, Zola's decision to juxtapose an old woman who cannot speak with a cat who seemingly can makes perfect sense. By depicting our proneness to language loss, Zola aims to remind us just how easily *homo loquens* can succumb to a state of mute animality.[49]

"menacé d'aphasie"

The next literary figure in this study, Marcel Proust, needed no reminders of this fragility of language, nor of the devastating effects of stroke. In 1903, his father Adrien Proust, one of France's most prominent physicians, suffered a brain hemorrhage while serving on a thesis committee at his Medical School. He died 3 days later, with his son Marcel at his bedside. Two years after that, in September 1905, Proust's mother Jeanne developed acute aphasia and paralysis resulting from uremia (kidney failure). She died 2 days after the onset of these symptoms. Her paralysis, together with her sudden inability to speak, left her son to wonder in letters to friends, "what she thought and what she suffered."[50] It is well known that Proust based the illness and death of Marcel's grandmother in the *Recherche* directly on his own mother's last days. In Part 1 of *The Guermantes Way*, Marcel's grandmother begins to suffer from uremic trouble, which causes her vision to deteriorate, then her hearing, her mobility, and finally her speech: "her pain grew less, but the impediment in her speech increased. We were obliged to ask her to repeat almost everything she said. And now my grandmother, realizing that we could no longer understand her, gave up altogether the attempt to speak and lay perfectly still."[51] Exactly like Madame Raquin, the face of Marcel's grandmother is said to be "grave and stony, her hands motionless on the sheet," and her inability at one point to recognize her grandson is attributed by the family doctor Cottard to the very same illness that afflicts Fouan in *La Terre*, namely, a "congestion of the brain" [congestion du cerveau].[52] According to recent biographers like William C. Carter and the historian of neurology Julien Bogousslavsky, this scene represents one of several pieces of evidence of the profound and lingering effect that Jeanne Proust's loss of speech had on her then 34-year-old son. For the rest of his life, Proust was beset with a pathological fear of losing his speech, a fear he once described in an essay he wrote on Baudelaire as being "terrorized by aphasia" [menacé d'aphasie].[53]

This aphasiaphobia would suddenly grow worse in 1917 when Proust began to experience symptoms of memory loss, facial palsy, and speech troubles. His speech became generally slurred, probably due to his abuse of veronal and other barbiturates. He also noticed himself uttering more and more paraphasias, and he found certain words difficult or even impossible to pronounce. Convinced these were the first signs of the same brain disease that had taken both his parents, Proust consulted his mother's neurologist Joseph Babinski. Like Samuel Johnson, Proust was a man who was prone to self-diagnosis, and it was not uncommon for him to arrive at his doctor's office with a plan for treatment already formulated. In this instance, the extreme solution Proust proposed to Dr Babinski was trepanation, or the boring of a hole into his skull. Babinski dissuaded Proust against such a radical procedure and managed to reassure him that his language faculty was still intact by having him pronounce various tongue twisters like *constantinopolitain* and *artilleur de l'artillerie*.[54] Still, this frightening firsthand experience with speech trouble also found its way into the *Recherche* through the character of Bergotte, who undergoes similar symptoms in the very same section of *The Guermantes Way* where Marcel describes his grandmother's aphasia. Bergotte's illness is unknown to Marcel, rendered as a matter of gossip and conjecture: "he was very ill, some people said with albuminuria, like my grandmother, while according to others he had a tumour."[55] Whether the writer's health troubles stem from his kidneys or a brain tumor, "He was now quite blind, and often he even had trouble with his speech" [sa parole meme s'embarrassait souvent].[56] Below we will examine other less personal renderings of speech trouble throughout the *Recherche*, specifically, the detailed case of the Baron de Charlus, who suffers a stroke and resulting aphasia in *Time Regained*. Before that, however, we must clarify first, the extent and the source of Proust's familiarity with neurology and aphasiology, and second, the major developments in the area of speech pathology from the period of Broca to the early twentieth century that inform those scenes from the *Recherche* depicting language loss or breakdown.

With a celebrated doctor for a father, and his brother Robert a prominent doctor as well, Proust grew up in a household steeped in the medical ideas of the day. His father was friends with most of Europe's leading neurologists, doctors like Joseph Babinksi, Jules Déjérine, and Charcot's star pupil, Edouard Brissaud. Proust would be treated by all of these men at different points in his life, and Brissaud, who founded the *Revue Neurologique* in 1893, later served as the model for the character of Dr Du Boulbon in the *Recherche*.[57] While Proust's medical background would be even further expanded from an early age, owing to his lifelong troubles with asthma, Julien Bogoussalvsky still insists that the interest in neurological disorders seen throughout the *Recherche* did not begin in earnest until the death of Adrien Proust in 1903: "Proust first heard of neurological diseases from his father who, while still in training, had worked at times under the influence of Charcot, who had conducted studies on stroke, aphasia, hysteria, and neurasthenia. These studies were well known to Marcel Proust. However, it is noteworthy that it is only after his father's death in 1903 that Proust's interest in neurology and neurologists increased."[58] As further evidence of this clinical turning point for Proust's writing, Bogousslavsky cites Proust's decision shortly after his father's death to write "a book about doctors."[59] Another statement Proust would later make to his caretaker Céleste Albaret attests to the impact of Adrien Proust's death on the direction of the project that began as *Jean Santeuil*. "When one is a doctor's son," Proust told Albaret, "one ends up becoming one as well. . . . I am more a doctor than the doctors."[60] The question, then, is exactly what kind of "doctor" the influence of his father would lead him to become.

Adrien Proust's prestige in the French medical establishment came primarily from his groundbreaking work on hygiene and the controlling of epidemics, but he also researched and published extensively on neurological and aphasiological disorders. In all likelihood, Marcel Proust got the idea for trepanation from a work his father had written on the very same subject, his 1874 study *L'aphasie et la trepanation* (1874), which assessed the possible benefits of trepanation in treating language loss. Adrien Proust's most important contribution to the field of aphasiology, his 1872 study *L'aphasie*, stressed the "diverse varieties of aphasia," by combining the available data from the famous cases of Broca and Trousseau together with his own firsthand observations of aphasic patients at the Hôpital de la Charité in 1871.[61] Despite its many merits, Dr Proust's *L'aphasie* is a mostly forgotten text in the history of aphasiology. Nevertheless, *L'aphasie* is arguably the most interesting (and overlooked within Proust Studies) source-text when it comes to speech and language disturbances in the *Recherche*. Dr Proust's study begins in modest fashion with an attempt to clarify and delimit the nomenclature of aphasiology. Aphasiological terms, he felt, had become increasingly occluded for reasons that will sound quite familiar to readers of Marcel Proust:

> But herein lies the difficulty. It is caused by the arbitrariness of the definitions. We use aphasia to refer to any trouble or alteration of speech, whatever the cause. And aphasia ceases to be a symptom, a distinct condition. It is no more than a word, serving to categorize a series of symptoms that have in common a difficulty with the articulation of language.[62]

Although Dr Proust insists that it is not his intention to engage in "some obscure metaphysical dissertation" and that he will simply state "clear and evident facts," he embarks on a much more general, philosophical discussion of the nature of consciousness, of exterior versus interior forms of language, and of the relationship between language and memory, all in a style full of proto-Proustian digressions which undoubtedly stretch the genre conventions of the medical case study.[63]

In order to clarify his technical point about nomenclature, Dr Proust distinguishes between two main forms of language, what he calls "natural language" (or "langage d'action") and "artificial language."[64] The first of these forms is said to include any and all bodily movements that signify something, whether thoughts, feelings, intentions, etc. This natural type of body language, Dr Proust notes, is something that we share with other animals, and it includes both voluntary and involuntary gestures, so long as they indicate some state of being to another party. Although this natural expressiveness of the body can be "as eloquent as speech itself," it does not suffice to render the subtler nuances of thought and emotion.[65] Therefore, another type of language is necessary for man to fully express himself. This second order of language Dr Proust calls "artificial," not because of its intrinsic character, which he insists is just as natural as body language, but because it relies on the use of "conventional signs."[66] In line with Broca, Dr Proust provides case after case to disprove the common misconceptions that aphasia is caused by paralysis or intellectual impairment. The ultimate conclusion his casework leads him to is that of a separation between thought (or consciousness) and language. For him, the demonstrable intelligence of his patients indicates that consciousness must exist in some manner apart from the faculty of language:

> It has been proven, I believe, by these experiments, that it is neither the impairment of intelligence, nor the impairment of word-memory which prevents aphasics from expressing themselves, from making their thoughts, their feelings, their wishes, understood through language. All the experts have remarked that in the case of aphasics, a lesion to the intelligence is never sufficient to explain their language trouble. Aphasics have more than enough intelligence for speaking. But some have argued aphasia is a type of verbal amnesia. Our experiments prove that it is no such thing.[67]

In addition to arguing against the common misconception that aphasia was an intellectual impairment, Dr Proust also rejects the theory that aphasia involves an impairment of memory. This view of language loss as word-amnesia, which did hold some currency in the 1870s and 1880s, was rejected by many other aphasiologists, including Désiré Bernard, in his *De L'aphasie* (1889), and later on by Marcel Proust's uncle Henri Bergson in *Matter and Memory* (1896). Although Dr Proust admits the difficulty of differential diagnosis between aphasia and word-amnesia in those cases where the available vocabulary is small and haltingly produced, the counterevidence presented by the various forms of copious aphasia he observed (along with the ability of so many aphasics to understand words spoken to them) forces him to conclude that the word-amnesia view must be abandoned. Just as thought and language are ultimately separate for him, so too are the faculties of word-recall and word-articulation. To know a word, he reminds us, is not necessarily to be able to use it.

"dissonant voices"

Many of Adrien Proust's concerns in *L'aphasie* clearly prefigure the reflections on language made by Marcel in the *Recherche*. With Proust-père, Proust-fils would come to share a fascination with nomenclature, the distinction between natural and conventional sign systems (or Cratylism vs. Hermogenism), and the relation between language and memory. Most importantly, Marcel Proust shared with his father a desire to exhaustively catalog the diverse forms and causes of language breakdown. Adrien Proust's contributions to the field of aphasiology came at a time when the cerebral basis of language and language loss had become a kind of dogma in European medical circles. Although Broca would lose the battle over the most appropriate name for this new pathology to Armand Trousseau, there was little debate when Adrien Proust wrote *L'aphasie* over the fundamental principle of cerebral localization. After the studies of Monsieurs Tan and Lelong, Broca continued to compile case after case in support of his theory, so that by the Spring of 1863, he could already boast 25 more examples of aphemia coinciding with lesions to the left frontal lobe. The result, as L. S. Jacyna notes in *Lost Words*, was that, "by 1865 the notion that there was a cerebral basis for the faculty of language had achieved the status of an orthodoxy; there were few who would dispute its status as a scientific 'fact.' Those who would not recognize this were fit for scorn."[68] Not surprisingly then, in 1874, when an unknown 26-year-old medical assistant from the Psychiatric Institute in Breslau purported to have discovered not only an alternate language center but also an altogether different form of aphasia corresponding to it, it sent shock waves through the field of aphasiology.

Carl Wernicke's *The Aphasia Symptom-Complex: A Psychological Study on an Anatomical Basis* (1874) offered both a corrective and an expansion of the aphasic syndrome. Whereas Broca had relied on the invariability of symptoms from case to case as proof of the distinctness of his pathology, Wernicke took the opposite approach. Like Adrien Proust, Wernicke stressed instead "the variability in the clinical picture of aphasia."[69] All of Broca's aphemic patients had two features in common: their auditory comprehension remained intact, but their vocabularies when speaking could be limited in some cases to as little as a single word (e.g. "tan" or Baudelaire's "cré nom"). The majority of

Wernicke's patients presented with an exactly opposite symptomatology. The working vocabularies of these patients, though often marred by neologistic jargon, still remained significantly larger than the aphemic patients of Broca. Their ability to comprehend language, on the other hand, was profoundly disturbed. For the typical case of this new language disorder, Wernicke writes: "Many words were spontaneously used correctly, but in contrast, only a few were comprehended well, and these only with great difficulty."[70] The presence of jargon, or spontaneous nonsense language, in so many cases meant that Wernicke had to combat a very different misdiagnosis from the one Broca had worked to correct a decade earlier.[71] While Broca had been more concerned about the misdiagnoses of diminished intelligence or paralysis in his patients, the verbal behavior of Wernicke's patients easily lent itself to "erroneous interpretations of such symptoms as dementia by experienced and intelligent physicians."[72] Like his predecessor, Wernicke was able to support his clinical findings with postmortem anatomical evidence. In the majority of cases, the lesion site was not to be found in Broca's area, but in a posterior section of the temporal lobe that would soon come to be known as Wernicke's area. Based on these pre- and postmortem findings, Wernicke concluded that "the great variability of the clinical picture of aphasia moves between the two extremes of pure motor aphasia and the pure sensory form. The demonstration of these two types must be regarded as conclusive proof of the existence of two anatomically separate language centers."[73] Variability of symptom and cause, though still understood in the anatomical terms of lesion sites, now became the revised dogma of aphasiology.

In the decades that followed the work of Paul Broca, Adrien Proust, Carl Wernicke et al., the stakes of their cumulative research gradually became apparent to scholars not only in the sciences, but also from more humanistic fields such as philosophy, literature, and psychology. The theory of cerebral localization served, according to Jacyna, "as the occasion for a confrontation between two worldviews that had vied for supremacy in France throughout the nineteenth century. At issue between them was the question of whether the distinction between spirit and matter, mind and body, was inviolable or whether the former categories should be collapsed into the latter."[74] This debate held dramatic consequences for both theological and humanist understandings of the nature of man and of his most defining faculty of language. Would finding a material basis for language close the gap, already threatened by Darwinism, between man and animal? Would a purely anatomical understanding of language be the last step down a slippery slope which ended in the denial of God and the discarding of the Soul?[75] In direct response to this crisis, a major schism occurred on these issues between two camps beginning in the late nineteenth century. As Jacyna demonstrates in Chapter 6 of *Lost Words*, both camps acknowledged the ever-increasing variety of the clinical picture of speech and language disorders, however, their views on etiology and methodology were vastly opposed. The first of these two camps remained staunchly materialist, and they were eventually dubbed the "diagram-makers" for their strict adherence to schematic maps and models of brain-processing. The second camp became known as the "holists" or "iconoclasts" for the challenges they put to what had by the 1890s become the orthodoxy of neurolinguistics. The first of these "dissonant voices," to borrow Jacyna's term for them, was the English aphasiologist John Hughlings Jackson (1835–1911).[76] What distinguished Hughlings Jackson's approach and made him such a controversial figure during the heyday of the diagram-makers was the equal weight he placed on psychological factors for any full understanding of disordered speech. Henri Bergson would also offer a sustained critique of the baldly materialist view of language and the increasingly elaborate schemata of the diagram-makers in his 1896 work *Matter and Memory*. Among these many dissonant voices, however, the most important figure for this study is certainly Sigmund Freud, whose influence on the issue of language breakdown is first felt in the works of Proust. Over the next three chapters as well, we will see how the Freudian view would come to dominate literary representations of speech and language disorders for almost a century.

The psychopathological account of language disturbance is most often associated with Freud's 1904 text *The Psychopathology of Everyday Life*, but it was much earlier, in his lesser-known 1891 work *On Aphasia: A Critical Study*, that Freud laid the groundwork for his psychogenic theories on verbal anomalies such as anomia, perseveration, paraphasia, and parapraxis.[77] In *On Aphasia*, Freud seconds many of the reservations first made by Hughlings Jackson with respect to the diagram-makers. Freud critiques their reductionist account of language as an anatomical process involving discrete centers, arguing instead for a more holistic speech apparatus which integrates several different processes throughout the brain: "the significance of the factor of localization for aphasia has been overrated, and . . . we should be well advised once again to concern ourselves with the functional states of the apparatus of speech."[78] According to Freud, the diagram-makers had pushed their anatomical approach to the point of a *reductio ad absurdum*, with new symptoms being linked to increasingly circumscribed lesion sites. Here again the vital importance of this issue of language breakdown, well beyond the field of speech pathology, becomes apparent. In the 1890s, debates over the etiology of aphasia also had far-reaching implications for fields like the one Freud was about to found. In this respect, Freud's rejection of the strictly anatomical etiology of aphasia in this early text is probably best understood as an act of self-preservation. Clearly, Freud foresees the threat posed by their radical materialism for the future of psychoanalysis, and he already begins to assert the relevance of the psyche to these questions in *On Aphasia.* He also begins to blur the dividing line between aphasic disturbances and the kinds of disturbance found in otherwise healthy patients:

> the paraphasia observed in aphasic patients does not differ from the incorrect use and the distortion of words which the healthy person can observe in himself in states of fatigue or divided attention or under the influence of disturbing affects—the kind of thing that frequently happens to our lecturers and causes the listener painful embarrassment.[79]

These everyday forms of disturbance are crucial to the direction speech pathology takes in the early twentieth century, simply put, because they can occur without any lesion to the brain. By calling attention to these more marginal forms of language breakdown, Freud allows for etiologies other than the strictly anatomical one offered by the diagram-makers. In the process, he preserves a role for the Psyche in the production of language, and he takes the first step toward the more elaborate psychogenic account of language disturbance he would develop in *The Psychopathology of Everyday Life.*

In his *Psychopathology*, Freud deals with many of the same verbal anomalies Proust catalogs in the *Recherche*, common mistakes in speech such as the forgetting of proper names, slips of the tongue, substitutions, but also more pathological conditions such as anomia, echolalia, and stuttering. Rather than a neurogenic account of these conditions, what Freud offers instead is a psychogenic reading of different types of speech disturbance. In each and every case, some unconscious drive such as repression or self-criticism is said to *motivate* the mistake in speech. In this way, the idea of impairment in psychopathology is less simplistic than the one that typically comes with neurology, where a faculty either functions properly or does not function at all. Instead, one finds linguistic impairment understood in more gradual terms, and language breakdown is understood in terms of one faculty *actively* working to impede another. For example, in his famous auto-diagnosis of his own forgetting of names, Freud writes: "I can no longer conceive the forgetting of the name Signorelli as an accidental occurrence. I must recognize in this process the influence of a *motive*. There were motives which actuated the interruption in the communication of my thoughts."[80] Obviously, these motives are not thought to be actuated by an anatomical lesion. In a later chapter "On the Forgetting of Names and Order of Words," Freud revisits the anatomical view he first critiqued in *On Aphasia*. Again, he asserts that a cause for the forgetting of proper names should not be sought "in circulatory or functional disturbances of the brain."[81] These complex processes are understood better, albeit more nebulously, as the experience of being "robbed by an unknown psychic force of the control over the proper names belonging to my memory."[82] In cases of embarrassing verbal slips, where one word is substituted for another, he argues that there is present an unconscious force of "self-criticism, an internal contradiction against one's own utterance, which causes the speech blunder."[83] Similarly, with pathologies like stammering and stuttering which disrupt the rhythm of speech, Freud argues that the same unconscious mechanisms are at work: "here, as in the former cases, it is the inner conflict that is betrayed to us through the disturbance in speech."[84] The more polemical aspects of this new etiology will become clearer in Chapter 2, through debates over the cause of shell shock during World War I, but first it remains to lay out the role that speech disorders play in the *Recherche* and to show how Proust's portrayal of aphasia reflects the neurogenic/psychogenic schism outlined above.

"whispered words"

Proust was well accustomed to thinking about physical illness in psychopathological terms ever since the onset of his asthma around 1880. It was Adrien Proust who first diagnosed his son's breathing difficulties as a case of neurasthenia. The diagnosis of neurasthenia for asthmatic symptoms is significant in this context because it reflects the attitude of late-nineteenth-century medical science, where neurology and psychology were beginning to negotiate their discrete areas of expertise as well as their possible interrelations. As Bogousslavky and others have noted, in the 1880s, asthma was regularly understood in the same terms as hysteria, that is to say, it was treated as a nervous condition stemming from psychosomatic or neurasthenic causes. As such, young Marcel Proust's asthma was thought to straddle the body and the psyche. The representation of language breakdown in the *Recherche* reflects a similar dual etiology that acknowledges both neurological and psychological factors for a variety of speech and language disorders ranging from minor tics and malapropisms to stuttering, lisps, and aphasiological conditions such as anomia. Like Zola, Proust understood the novelistic project in explicitly medical terms, yet unlike Zola, his clinical viewpoint is not so rigidly materialist. If the Zola of *La Terre* can be called "the first post-Broca novelist," then Proust in the same way represents the first novelist of that generation represented by John Hughlings Jackson, Sigmund Freud, and Henri Bergson, all of whom sought to preserve the psyche against the materialist implications of cerebral localization.

The case of the Baron de Charlus is the best example of Proust's dual neuro/psycho-genic approach to language breakdown. Over the course of the *Recherche*, Charlus undergoes a sort of linguistic downfall, from his initial position as the greatest talker of the social world Marcel inhabits to a frail aphasic who can only "pronounce certain words with difficulty and incorrectly."[85] Marcel does not learn that Charlus has been convalescing "after an attack of apoplexy" until that late scene in *Time Regained* when he is on his way to the party of the Princess de Guermantes and notices Charlus in his cab, being cared for, "like a child," by Charlus' former lover Jupien:

Jupien helped the Baron to descend and I greeted him. He spoke to me very rapidly, in a voice so inaudible that I could not distinguish what he was saying, which wrung from him, when for the third time I made him repeat his remarks, a gesture of impatience that astonished me by its contrast with the impassivity which has face had at first displayed, which was no doubt an aftereffect of his stroke. But when after a while I had grown accustomed to this pianissimo of whispered words, I perceived that the sick man retained the use of his intelligence absolutely intact. There were, however, two M. de Charluses, not to mention any others. Of the two, one, the intellectual one, passed his time in complaining that he suffered from progressive aphasia, that he constantly pronounced one word, one letter by mistake for another.[86]

What is most striking about this passage is the explicit, even self-conscious, way in which it rehearses Adrien Proust's point about the intelligence of aphasics remaining intact. At first glance, the symptomatology described during this encounter easily lends itself to a neurophysiological viewpoint. Marcel stresses the Baron's partial paralysis, for which he requires Jupien's assistance. As in the case of Madame Raquin, we are told of the "impassivity" of Charlus' face and the "painful effort he had to make to move his arm."[87] There is the hint of paralysis to the speech organs (or apraxia) as well, in the feebleness of Charlus' "pianissimo of whispered words" [pianissimo de parole susurrées].[88] The actual transcribed speech of Charlus in the scene, though inaudible and full of erroneous substitutions, is still fairly copious, placing him closer to a diagnosis of Wernicke's aphasia than to Broca's.[89] Altogether, from his progressive aphasia to his paralytic gait, Charlus represents to Marcel a classic case of "that lack of co-ordination which follows upon maladies of the spinal column and the brain."[90] In short, an attack of apoplexy has produced a lesion, which in turn has produced an anomic disturbance to the language faculty with possible apraxia further enfeebling Charlus' voice. From the very next sentence, however, the narrator's diagnosis shifts entirely to the realm of the psychogenic:

But as soon as he actually made such a mistake, the other M. de Charlus, the subconscious one, who was as desirous of admiration as the first was of pity and out of vanity did things that the first would have despised, immediately,

like a conductor whose orchestra has blundered, checked the phrase which
he had started and with infinite ingenuity made the end of his sentence
follow coherently from the word which he had in fact uttered by mistake for
another but which he thus appeared to have chosen. Even his memory was
intact, and from it his vanity impelled him, not without the fatigue of the
most laborious concentration, to drag forth this or that ancient recollection,
of no importance, which concerned myself and which would demonstrate to
me that he had preserved or recovered all his lucidity of mind.[91]

Here again the influence of Adrien Proust is felt through the implicit rejection
of the word-amnesia theory of language loss. The psychogenic view underlying
this second passage takes two main forms. First, there is the suggestion of a
split self within Charlus, one side of which actively redirects the verbal output
of his other intellectual or conscious self. Within the orchestral conceit Proust
creates to describe this elaborate process, Charlus' damaged brain would seem
to correspond to the blundering orchestra, in which case the conductor would
then represent some psychic force which, in Freudian terms, *motivates* these
verbal substitutions. The issue of intention in this passage is therefore extremely
complex as well. Charlus is said to consciously intend some initial word, but
when his brain then unintentionally produces the wrong word, this psychic
force overrides the initial conscious intention, improvising a kind of second-
order meaning out of these mistakes in speech. The other obvious psychogenic
dimension to this passage comes in the suggestion of nonanatomical causes for
Charlus' speech blunders: the presence of fatigue in an old man which partially
diminishes his ability to retrieve the *mot juste* and the emotional disturbance
that drives Charlus nevertheless to go on speaking more and more forcefully
as the scene progresses. Both of these factors gesture toward a Freudian
psychopathology in which everyday states such as fatigue or emotional distress
can alter or diminish the otherwise normal function of the speech apparatus.
The longer Marcel tries to understand these "whispered words," the more he
vacillates between the physical and psychical interpretations of their cause:

my ears soon accustomed themselves to his pianissimo. The sound had in
any case, I think, gradually grown in volume while the Baron was speaking,
perhaps because the weakness of his voice was due in part to a nervous
apprehension which was dispelled when he was distracted by the presence

of another person and ceased to think about it, though possibly, on the other hand, the feeble voice corresponded to the real state of his health and the momentary strength with which he spoke in conversation was the result of an artificial, transient and even dangerous excitement.[92]

Here Marcel adds yet another everyday cause, distractedness, to the list of nonanatomical factors that might be affecting the volume, tonality, and accuracy of Charlus' speech. It should also be noted that the three alternative causes Marcel suggests—emotion, fatigue, and distraction—are the very same triggers for paraphasia cited above by Freud. In *On Aphasia*, Freud argued that "in states of fatigue or divided attention or under the influence of disturbing affects," aphasics, just like otherwise healthy persons, can undergo additional disturbances in speech from a psychogenic cause that is wholly unrelated to their anatomical lesion.[93]

This depiction of "progressive aphasia" pushes our history forward from the clinically crude portraits of language loss by Zola in several important ways, through its complex and sometimes conflicted mixture of medical diagnosis with psychological observation. This aphasic portrayal from *Time Regained* is not, however, the first moment when Marcel notices a profound disruption to the speech patterns of the Baron. Much earlier in *The Captive*, Marcel observes the first signs of Charlus' aging through changes to his speech, during that long party hosted by the Verdurins where Charlus is eventually betrayed by his lover Morel: "one could tell that M. de Charlus had aged from wholly different signs, such as the extraordinary frequency in his conversation of certain expressions that had taken root in it and used now to crop up at every moment (for instance: 'the concatenation of circumstances') and upon which the Baron's speech leaned in sentence after sentence as upon a necessary prop."[94] For Marcel, the overreliance on certain stock phrases is indicative of a weakening or a partial loss of control over what was once the Baron's unsurpassed gift for witty repartee. This loss of control coincides with that phase in Charlus' life where he becomes increasingly unable or unwilling to conceal his homosexuality, and for Marcel, these two changes in the man are fundamentally linked. Linguistically, the problem this poses is exactly opposite to that of his eventual aphasic disturbance. Whereas Charlus will later struggle to vocalize any words at all, during the Verdurins' party, he repeatedly outs himself due to his inability

to *restrain* his speech. While scrutinizing the slightest of changes to Charlus'
intonation, his gestures, along with his many scandalous admissions, Marcel
becomes especially preoccupied with the question of etiology. What exactly
is provoking the Baron to risk social ruination? Marcel goes on to propose
a number of possible causes for these related losses of control, including the
effect of "a debauched life betrayed by moral degeneration" or "the senility of a
mind less capable than in the past of controlling its reflexes."[95] He also attempts
to identify a common pathological trait among older homosexuals, what he
calls "the manner that men of the Charlus type, whatever they may say, are
compelled to adopt when they have reached a certain stage in their malady,
just as sufferers from general paralysis or locomotor ataxia inevitably end by
displaying certain symptoms."[96] Obviously the compulsive verbal output that
accompanies this mysteriously psychosexual malady would fall under the
heading of an involuntary tic, rather than any neurological disorder.

The climax to this party scene, when Charlus is publicly rebuffed by his
lover Morel, offers an interesting counterpoint to the neurological account of
Charlus' state in *Time Regained*. Earlier in the party, Monsieur and Madame
Verdurin have conspired to dupe Morel into believing that Charlus has been
slandering the violinist's reputation in the highest social circles of Paris. Later
on, when Charlus approaches his lover, Morel openly accuses him of trying to
pervert him. Long familiar with the Baron's sadistic tendencies, Marcel braces
himself for the tirade he expects Charlus to unleash on both Morel and his
conspirators, but Charlus' response is altogether different: "an extraordinary
thing happened. M. de Charlus stood speechless [muet], dumbfounded,
measuring the depths of his misery without understanding its cause, unable to
think of a word to say, raising his eyes to gaze at each of the company in turn,
with a questioning, outraged, suppliant air, which seemed to be asking them
not so much what had happened as what answer he ought to make."[97] Just
as before, Marcel endeavors to pinpoint a root cause, now for Charlus' total
lack of reaction, and he struggles to understand what it is about this acute
emotional shock that induces an almost catatonic state in the Baron for the
remainder of the scene. As he describes the furious response he had expected,
Marcel rehashes the very same discourse of neurotic enervation that structures
Thérèse Raquin. Terms like *sensitif*, *nerveux*, and even *hystérique* are used to

explicate the neurotic temperament of the Baron as well as his usual response to this type of affront.[98] The great irony of this scene is that this emotionally traumatic event produces virtually identical symptoms in Charlus to those of his later aphasic episode: "this great nobleman . . . could do nothing, in the paralysis of his every limb as well as his tongue, but cast around him terror-stricken, suppliant, bewildering glances outraged by the violence that was being done to him. In a situation so cruelly unforeseen, this great talker could do no more than stammer" [ce grand discoureur ne sut que balbutier].[99] Examined together, these moments of language breakdown suggest that Charlus has been undergoing a "progressive aphasia" for quite some time, although the sense of aphasia in this case is as much metaphorical as clinical. Charlus, after all, is not only the great talker of the *Recherche*, the master of eloquence, but he is also the novel's supreme expert in nomenclature. Charlus, better than anyone else, better even than the pedantic Brichot, knows the names of things. Because of this, Marcel expresses a wish that the Baron would have taken up the practice of writing, only a few pages before he notes those first signs of aging in Charlus' speech: "he would have performed a rare service by writing, for, while he observed and distinguished everything, he also knew the name of everything he distinguished. . . . If he had written books, even bad ones . . . what a delightful dictionary, what an inexhaustible inventory they would have been been!"[100] This detail of the Baron's dictionary-like knowledge of the names of things adds another layer of poignancy to his linguistic downfall. The sense of anomia here becomes twofold as well, indicating both a distinct pathological state and a more general fragility inherent to language itself.

The man who begins the *Recherche* by representing the greatest possible command over spoken language thus ends with the least. In a final indignity, he is silently reproached by the Duchess de Letourville for attending the party after she hears the Baron struggle to speak. Between these two poles represented by Charlus—the perfectibility of language versus its susceptibility to total breakdown—Proust provides us with a virtually comprehensive encyclopedia of other speech anomalies or defects of language. In his essay, "Proust and Indirect Language," Gerard Genette refers to the product of this encyclopedic task as the "essentially verbal universe of the *Recherche*."[101] Genette catalogs those characters who exist solely as silhouettes for the idiosyncratic speech patterns they exemplify. Characters like the Balbec Manager, with his many humorous malapropisms stand, in Genette's words, simply as "collections of the accidents of speech" [collections d'accidents de langage].[102] Along with the hotel manager, we might also include more clinically recognizable conditions like the stutters of Saniette and M. Verdurin (who despite his own stammer, cruelly mocks Saniette's speech impediment in *Sodom and Gomorrah*), and the pronounced lisp of Bréauté. There are also the various mispronunciations of words. Some are owed only to a lack of education, as in the case of Françoise or Bloch. Others, for Marcel, are less easily explained, for instance why the Liftboy, "who heard people, fifty times a day, calling for the 'lift' should never himself call it anything but a 'liff.'"[103] In *Time Regained*, he reflects back on these and all the other forms of linguistic deformity, bastardization, and breakdown of which he has taken note, and he observes of himself that these phenomena came to interest him so much that he altered the very way in which he listens to others: "the stories that people told escaped me, for what interested me was not what they were trying to say but the manner in which they said it and the way in which this manner revealed their character or their foibles."[104] In the end, what the manner of saying reveals to him is not the insights of neurology, but those of psychology: "a collection of psychological laws in which the actual purport of the remarks of each guest occupied but a very small space."[105] In the following chapter, we will see how these psychological laws of disordered speech were brought into even greater prominence during World War I.

Speech Disorders and Shell Shock in World War I Writing

"Shall I mutter and stutter and wangle my ticket
Or try another flutter and go back and stick it?"

– Wilfred Owen, from *The Hydra*

"Kindred Disorders"

The First World War was a watershed moment for speech pathology, as thousands of new cases of brain wounds and war neurosis (or "shell shock") rapidly increased medical knowledge as well as public awareness of resulting conditions like aphasia, stammering, and mutism.[1] This new level of public visibility meant that from the War years through the 1920s, the archetype of the aphasic, the stammerer, or the mute was now the soldier back from the trenches. The most comprehensive set of case studies on aphasia caused by head wounds to soldiers serving at the Front was compiled by the British neurologist Sir Henry Head (1861–1940). At the outbreak of the War, Head had shifted his attention away from his private practice to participate in the War effort by tending to wounded soldiers at the London Hospital. The experience of treating dozens of aphasic soldiers over a period of several years would inspire Head to publish his case studies, as part of his massive two-volume work *Aphasia and Kindred Disorders of Speech* (1926). Together, these reports provide an overview of the ongoing speech difficulties faced by many soldiers years after the War was over. Head's reports also offer a graphic and clinically exact account of the types of head wounds from which soldiers were now able to survive, owing to medical advances and improved training of combat medics. Among the 16 reports of War-related aphasia Head published (listed as Patients 1–19), 10 were caused by bullets entering the brain. Three other cases were caused by shrapnel from shell casings penetrating the skull. Patient 10 was left severely aphasic from a hand grenade blast, Patient 2 was kicked by his horse, and Patient 19 was bombed from an airplane while riding his motorcycle.

This unique combination of circumstances—the scale of the War itself and technological increases in firepower, both coupled paradoxically with higher survival rates from head wounds—gave Head the opportunity to study an entirely new type of aphasic patient, one who was still young and able-bodied enough to recover. Fifty years earlier, Broca's work had also benefited greatly by a certain type of access, namely, pre- and postmortem access to patients like Monsieur Tan and Lelong. He had been able to subject them to exhaustive neurological and physiological tests prior to their deaths. He was then able to confirm his hypotheses as to the precise location of their lesions upon autopsy. What Broca did not have the opportunity to study, however, was the aphasic in a state of regeneration, gradually recovering their speech, sometimes word by word over a period of days, months, or even years. In the chapter of *Aphasia and Kindred Disorders* where Head outlines his methods of examination, he explains the many advantages of this new type of patient:

> In civilian practice many of those who suffer from aphasia are old, broken down in health and their general intellectual capacity is diminished. Most of them are affected with arterial degeneration and in many the blood tension is greatly increased. Such patients are easily fatigued and are obviously unsuitable for sustained examination. But the war brought under our care young men who were struck down in the full pride of health. Many of them were extremely intelligent, willing and anxious to be examined thoroughly. As their wounds healed, they were encouraged and cheered by the obvious improvement in their condition. They were euphoric rather than depressed, and in every way contrasted profoundly with the state of the aphasic met with in civilian practice.[2]

Throughout both volumes of *Aphasia and Kindred Disorders*, one encounters this unexpectedly optimistic tone, about the young aphasic's higher chances of recovery as well as the benefits for science of access to this new type of patient.

Head even points out the relative "advantage" of bullet wounds over the types of lesions brought on by stroke, since the patient who survives being shot in the head tends to recover more speech function more rapidly.[3]

Head's entire approach to aphasiology can be summed up by his conviction that "No two examples of aphasia exactly resemble one another; each represents the response of a particular individual to the abnormal conditions."[4] This individualizing approach to disorders of speech is reflected from his theoretical writings to his treatment of his patients. It also informed his approach to the "genre" of the aphasiological case study.[5] In order to gauge each soldier's particular impairments, Head subjected them to a battery of verbal and cognitive tests, assessing their ability to name and recognize common objects, remember various facts and dates, and perform simple acts of arithmetic and symbolic thinking. To track their progress, he continued to retest some of his patients for up to 7 years after the War. Although he insisted on the need to treat each case on its own terms, Head still felt confident distinguishing between four roughly classed varieties of aphasic disorder: (1) Verbal, (2) Syntactical, (3) Nominal, and (4) Semantic.[6] Head's class of verbal aphasics spoke with varying degrees of fluency, but they all struggled to correctly form their words and phrases. Syntactical aphasics often spoke copiously, but they omitted connectors like prepositions, articles, and conjunctions, and they were regularly prone to jargon when attempting spontaneous speech. Nominal aphasics had difficulty recalling the names of things, categorical terms, nomenclature, etc. Lastly, semantic aphasics had difficulty understanding words in contexts other than their strictly verbal meaning.

One of Head's more severe cases will help to illustrate the extremes of impairment and improvement that characterized the new aphasic of the War generation. Patient 7 was a Scotch steelworker who had suffered a gunshot wound to the left hemisphere in 1917. Six weeks after the wound, Head reports that the man was still "so grossly aphasic that it was impossible to obtain from him any coherent information." Gradually, a diagnosis of nominal aphasia emerged as Patient 7 continued to struggle to produce nouns either spontaneously or by repetition, all while improving in other areas of speech. After 17 weeks, Patient 7 still could not produce many basic names for things, though Head notes that the sounds he did produce were increasingly close to the mark. Attempts to recall a word like "scissors," for instance, resulted in the sounds, "sis . . . sit, sitty, sizz." The color black was pronounced, "blat, berlat, blad." Trying to recall the months of the year also produced neologistic jargon. For February: "Fenchurch, Jan-jey, Jan-jey." For September: "Eps-ten, Ex-pent, Ex-pesnt. For October, "Ex, Ox, Ox, Ox-toe, Ox-tove."[7] It would take 4 years and 9 months before Patient 7 was finally able to pass Head's battery of tests, and though his anomia had shown dramatic improvement, he still spoke slowly and wrote with great difficulty.[8]

Soon after its publication, *Aphasia and Kindred Disorders* quickly became the most influential aphasiological text of its era, not just for the light it shed on the prevalence of speech disorders among soldiers returned from combat, but also, and perhaps primarily, for its critical overview of the history of aphasiological theories and methods. Head belonged firmly to the "holist" countertradition within aphasiology (outlined in Chapter 1), which believed that the theory of cerebral localization had become much too narrowly applied, resulting in an oversimplified understanding of what were extremely complex neurolinguistic functions. In fact, it was Head who first used the pejorative label of "diagram-makers" to describe the schematic approach of doctors like Bastian, Meynert, and Lichtheim. Head argued vehemently against what he felt were the misleading effects of their work for actual therapeutic practice.

Much like Freud in this regard, Head had been strongly influenced during his clinical training by the aphasiological writings of John Hughlings Jackson (1835–1911). In *Lost Words*, Jacyna notes the impact Hughlings Jackson's work would eventually have, via its assimilation and retransmission first by Freud (in 1891) and much later by Henry Head: "Head followed Hughling Jackson's lead and insisted on the necessity of understanding aphasic disorders as psychological as well as anatomical or merely behavioral phenomena. Indeed, he seemed to see such an emphasis upon the patient's subjective experience as one of the defining features of the new neurology that was emerging in the aftermath of the First World War."[9] This integration of psychology into the aphasiological examination had profound effects on the way Head applied his treatment method. As he stresses in his chapter on "Methods of Examination," the patient's reaction to the tests themselves was as vital to him as their performance: "It is particularly important to write down at the moment any statement which throws light on the ideas or feelings of the patient with regard to the test."[10] The overtones of a Freudian "talking cure" here are evident, and in several of the case studies, this concern for the patient's feelings steers Head toward the role of a psychoanalyst recording the traumatic memories as part of the patient's overall disturbance. Dealing with traumatic memories formed part of Head's attempt to broaden the scope of the aphasiological case study in order to arrive at what he calls in an earlier publication a "psychology of the concrete individual."[11] Ultimately, this entailed major changes to the genre conventions of the clinical case study, with an unusual emphasis on dialogism between doctor and patient, and above all, a diachronic narrative of each patient's life story and process of recovery. Head devoted hundreds of pages to detailing the particularities of his soldiers, beyond clinical descriptions of their wounds and their performances on tests. He also delved extensively into their backgrounds, their education, and their memories of the War. For this reason, Jacyna calls Head's critique of the diagrammatic style of case study, "in large part a trenchant literary criticism."[12]

"no stammer previous to shock"

This mixed method, derived from Hughlings Jackson, of combining anatomical knowledge with a psychologists' sensitivity to the personality and life experiences of the individual patient was also the hallmark of Head's friend and colleague, Dr W. H. R. Rivers (1864–1922), in dealing with another type of speech-impaired soldier. In his role as medical officer at the Craiglockhart War Hospital, Rivers dealt primarily with shell-shocked officers, many of whom suffered from profound disturbances of speech. Among the many officer-patients who stayed at Craiglockhart during the War were the poets Siegfried Sassoon and Wilfred Owen, the latter developing a slight stammer from shell shock. Later in this chapter, we will turn to the poetic response of Wilfred Owen to problems of voice related to his War experiences.

Head's dictum that no two aphasic cases were alike could certainly be applied to shell shock as well, and it would be almost oxymoronic to speak of the "typical" shell shock patient. Symptoms were so varied and conflicting that it made diagnosis of the condition extremely difficult for combat medics and physicians. Some soldiers developed paralysis in the arms or legs where no physical injury was present, whereas other soldiers would develop involuntary trembling in those same limbs. Some lost their hearing either partially or totally. Others lost their sight, again with no discernible physical cause. Partial amnesia, headaches, hallucinations, nightmares, and sleeplessness were all common as well. Lastly, a disturbance in the soldier's speech patterns was one of the most frequently occurring features of shell shock, and the varieties of disorder ranged from the mildest of stammers to a complete loss of the ability to speak. The terms "war stammering" and "war mutism" arose to denote this sudden onset of speech trouble with soldiers who, in almost every instance, had spoken fluently their entire lives but developed stammers or went totally mute in reaction to traumatic experiences at the Front. One such case involved a 21-year-old private treated for shell shock in April 1916 at a hospital in Rouen:

> Progress. Has improved by slow degrees. Speech returned but some extreme difficulty owing to great stammering and stuttering. His facial muscles all tremble more or less when he attempts to speak. The stammer is now almost away (he had no stammer previous to shock). Pains in head much less severe. Feet had improved greatly but are still numb to some extent and he has not attempted to stand.[13]

Many of the available case notes and medical reports reflect the diagnostic confusion of the time, as doctors, operating under the extreme pressures of Wartime medicine, struggled to treat a condition before it had been properly understood. As such, one detects a level of uncertainty in early casenotes of shell shock, where doctors suggest possible connections between seemingly unrelated symptoms. In the above case, for instance, the medical report indicates a strong relation between the speech trouble and the involuntary spasms of his facial muscles. Other reports often implicitly connect the silence of the mute soldier to their repression of traumatic memories, for instance, in the case of a rifleman known as W. B. who in 1915 suddenly recovered his speech, following a long period of silence:

> Sent home from Flanders May 1915, suffering from Shock (Shell) with symptoms of loss of memory, almost total, complete loss of speech, partial

loss of sight and hearing. Tremor sweating, sleeplessness, probably hallucinations of sight. Slow improvement til Oct 1915, when suddenly he received speech and for 72 hours he remembered about his time in Flanders, forgetting meanwhile all he knew of the Dublin University V.A.D. Hospital . . . where he was being cared for.[14]

Particularly during the War, discussions about shell shock were deeply fraught due to a conflict between the demands of the military, on the one hand, and the therapeutic goals of medical science, on the other. In his historical study of the treatments and debates surrounding the condition, *Shell Shock: Traumatic Neurosis and the British Soldiers of the First World War*, Peter Leese calls this a period of "confrontation between discipline and welfare," where the well-being of the patient often took second place to the requirements of manpower at the Front.[15] Consequently, treatment methods were geared less toward curing the patient than toward bringing symptoms under control in order to return the soldier to a "serviceable" state as quickly as possible. Moreover, since the question of a physical basis for shell shock had not yet been resolved, many military and medical figures spoke out against its validity as a disease.[16] Military authorities also expressed concern over the threat shell shock posed for general troop morale. The most cynical among them tied it to the problem of malingering, warning that if not carefully policed, shell shock would become the easiest way for a soldier to feign an inability to fight. For all of these reasons, as Leese explains, sufferers of this still-mystifying condition were subject to extreme levels of stigmatization:

> They sometimes offered outward visible signs of the war in a stutter or shuffling walk, but the damage of the war was mostly unseen, at first located in the brain, and later relocated to the psyche. Without bandages, scars or missing limbs, the shell shock casualty could not lay claim properly to a wound; without the prestige of a wound, he was under suspicion. In private his manhood could be doubted, in public his patriotism might be questioned.[17]

Shell-shocked soldiers and officers were acutely aware of the suspicions and stigmas that surrounded their condition. One of the only avenues available to them for voicing their own experiences came in the many hospital gazettes and literary magazines that sprung up during the War, such as *The Hydra*, the in-house magazine of Craiglockhart Hospital, which was edited by Wilfred Owen and premiered some of the war poetry of Siegfried Sassoon and others. As Leese shows, these hospital magazines offered a wide mix of attitudes on shell shock, ranging from propagandistic homilies about the patient's need to regather his wits and muster up the willpower to fight, to satirical editorials, cartoons, and poems by the soldiers themselves. In this context, the most relevant example is the poem "Just Shell Shock," published in the Springfield War Hospital Gazette in 1916. Like the majority of works that appeared in War hospital magazines, it was published under a pseudonym, "Gunner McPhail," and the poem offers a plainspoken reminder of how disorders of speech and hearing, however devastating, did not qualify as wounds deserving of recognition:

> Of course you've heard of shell shock
> But I don't suppose you think,
> What a wreck it leaves a chap
> After being in the pink . . .
> Or suppose you lose your speech, sir,
> Perhaps you're deaf and dumb as well,
> But you don't get no gold stripe to show,
> Although you've fought and fell[18]

A more canonical variation on the same theme is the poem "Survivors," written by Siegfried Sassoon in October 1917, during his stay at Craiglockhart War Hospital. Like the poem by McPhail, Sassoon's poem invokes the issue of war stammering explicitly, however, his manner of retaliating against the public stigma of shell shock is altogether different:

> No doubt they'll soon get well; the shock and strain
> Have caused their stammering, disconnected talk.
> Of course they're 'longing to go out again,' –
> These boys with old, scared faces, learning to walk.
> They'll soon forget their haunted nights; their cowed
> Subjection to the ghosts of friends who died, –
> Their dreams that drip with murder; and they'll be proud
> Of glorious war that shatter'd all their pride . . .

Men who went out to battle, grim and glad,
Children, with eyes that hate you, broken and mad.[19]

Whereas McPhail chooses to fire back at public opinion, from his privileged position as a shell shock victim, Sassoon instead ventriloquizes public opinion, relegating the voice of the actual soldier to a cliched quotation about how impatient they are to get back to the Front. Through this more satirically indirect approach, Sassoon reminds us first, how difficult it would be for the speech-impaired soldier to express the reality of shell shock, and second, how little weight their understanding of their own condition as patients would have carried at this time.

While pundits questioned the legitimacy of shell shock as a medical condition, neurologists and psychologists were busy seeking out its definitive cause. Debates on the etiology of shell shock hinged on the question of whether it had any physical basis to it or was a purely psychological reaction to traumatic combat experiences; in other words, whether it stemmed from trauma to the brain or to the psyche. Opinions split roughly along the same lines that we find in the field of aphasiology at the time, with neurogenic and psychogenic theories competing for dominance. The neurogenic (or organic) view held that shell shock was a type of concussive syndrome, or a form of nerve-exhaustion related to neurasthenia, in which the many impacts of combat did actual physical damage to the soldier's brain and nervous system, triggering various forms of war neurosis.[20] According to Leese, the neurogenic view was always in the minority, but it persisted throughout the War due to the high number of cases "on the borderline of concussion and neurosis," where soldiers had suffered both physical and psychic injuries, making differential diagnosis of psychic shock even more problematic.[21] With the rise of Freudianism in the 1920s, however, the psychogenic view would win out, and "shell shock" as a clinical designation would gradually be phased out in favor of the term "psycho-neurosis."[22]

The most official articulation of the psychogenic view of shell shock took place 2 months before the Armistice, in September 1918, at the Fifth Psycho-Analytical Congress in Budapest. Officials from the Central European Powers attended the event (mostly from concern over the problem of malingering) to hear leading psychoanalysts such as Sandor Ferenczi and Ernst Simmel give talks on the topic of war neurosis. Freud would later write the Introduction to their presentations, published together under the title *Psychoanalysis and the War Neuroses* (1919). Of all the participants, Ferenczi was arguably the most aggressive proponent of the psychogenic view, and in his talk, he used the topic as an opportunity to put neurologists in their place, so to speak: "The mass-experiment of the war has produced various severe neuroses, including those in which there could be no question of a mechanical influence, and the neurologists have likewise been forced to recognise that something was missing in their calculations, and this something was again—the psyche."[23] While many in the neurogenic camp had hearkened back to Hermann Oppenheim's research into the effects of trauma on the nervous system, proponents of the psychogenic view drew on Charcot's initial definition of hysteria, since shell shock bore an obvious resemblance to the model of hysteria in which the physical symptoms are said to occur where no underlying organic cause is present. For Ferenczi, shell shock was "like a museum of glaring hysterical symptoms" with "all the varieties of tic and shaking tremors, paralyses and contractures in monoplegic, hemiplegic and paraplegic forms, deafness and deaf and dumbness, stuttering and stammering, aphonia and rhythmical screaming."[24]

All participants of the Congress, of course, took their cue from Freud, who had explained war neurosis as a kind of "flight into disease" where the soldier embodies the threat to his life within himself as a new and separate "war-ego."[25] The various symptoms are then said to arise out of an ego-conflict whereby the older peace-time ego attempts to defend itself against the internalized threat of the war-ego.[26] Disturbances of speech occurring from shell shock were understood in these same terms, as a kind of defense mechanism against the terror of War. Thus, Ferenczi writes: "the symptoms of the terror, such as the immovable legs, the tremblings, the hesitating speech, seem to be useful automatisms; one is reminded by them of certain animals which simulate being dead when danger threatens."[27] As evidence for this theory, cases were cited of soldiers who developed mutism after having to play dead behind enemy lines or developed deaf-mutism as a reenactment of the traumatic memory of being buried alive in their trenches by explosions.

By the point at which Freud and his cohort had formulated the psychoanalytic account of war neurosis, the spectacle of shell shock had already expanded well beyond the confines of the War hospital and the psychiatric clinic into a common feature of everyday life on the homefront. All over Europe and Britain, millions of wounded and disfigured young men were a daily reminder of the consequences of the so-called Great War. But the shell-shocked soldier as well, marked by his shuffling gait and halting speech, became another reminder, albeit poorly understood, of the psychic effects of War.[28] Once the War had ended, and the shell-shocked soldier transitioned into the shell-shocked veteran, medical priorities shifted from the management of his symptoms to the assessment of his right to a disability pension. In his chapter on the complex medical politics behind the assessment of "disability" status for shell-shock victims, Leese outlines one telling case in which the Pension Board unanimously agreed that the soldier qualified for 100 percent disability owing solely to shell shock. The soldier, known as "Sapper O.," was assessed annually from 1917 to 1922, and his "progress" from year to year gives an insight into just how tenuous the recovery from traumatic war neurosis could be. In April 1918, a full year after he was declared too incapacitated for active service, his symptoms included "stutter, heartache, slight tremor, excited manner, dreams, sleeps badly." By June 1919, "stammer much improved," and 18 months later, in December 1920, there were "mild hand tremors, bad stammers, nervous, complains of headaches, palpitations, sweats, sinking feeling." But then, 4 years after he had seen active service, in December 1921, Sapper O's condition actually worsened: "stammering more than when enlisted, headaches, shaking and trembling on excitement." While Sapper O's case may not be a typical one, by virtue of its qualification for full disability pension, it does reveal that disordered speech was one of the most obdurate symptoms of war neurosis. In fact, many veterans retained the trace of a stammer for the rest of their lives.

"You can't communicate noise"

The poetic response to the War began as a response to an altogether different type of "failure" of language. One of the most common sentiments, expressed by virtually every World War I poet at some point, was a feeling of the indescribability (or unspeakability) of the War, a feeling that language was ultimately inadequate to the task of rendering the experience of trench warfare for those who hadn't fought in it themselves.[29] Their primary strategy for overcoming this different type of "failure" of language was to rely on an immediate and visually graphic diction, oftentimes violating rules of poetic decorum in the process, so as to immerse the reader as directly as possible in all the new horrible sights which had been made possible by the introduction of machine guns and heavy artillery into trench warfare. Hence the innumerable descriptions of the spectacle of corpses, both friend and foe, one encounters in poems and memoirs from the period. Because proximity to the enemy often made it too dangerous to bury the dead, soldiers would sometimes spend days sharing trenches with corpses, nicknaming them and even conversing with them in a macabre kind of coping mechanism, or simply staring for hours on end at their bluish faces. One of the most powerful examples of these new and traumatizing sights comes in *Goodbye to All That*, where Robert Graves matter-of-factly describes the first time he saw human brains, in a soldier who was not yet dead: "At my feet lay the cap he had worn, splashed with his brains. I had never seen human brains before; I somehow regarded them as a poetical figment."[30] In this context, one might also think of "Dulce et Decorum Est," in which the power of the poem is generally assumed to come from our being made to see, through the eyes of the speaker, the look of the man who fails to get his gas mask on in time, "the white eyes writhing in his face, / His hanging face, like a devil's sick of sin."[31]

That being said, the Great War was equally a war of noise—the steady bombardment of shells, the deafening machine-gun fire, the whizz of the sniper's bullet, the thumps of mortar cannons and grenades, the screams and moans of the wounded and the dying. It was, in other words, as much phonosagoria as phantasmagoria, an endless cacophony of new sounds that tested every soldier's nerves. In this respect, it would seem to be no accident that Graves begins his account of seeing the soldier's brain with a description of the sound the dying man was making, "a snoring noise mixed with animal groans."[32] Likewise, in "Dulce et Decorum Est," Owen devotes equal attention to the horrible sounds of the gassed soldier, first his "yelling," then his "guttering, choking, drowning," and finally the sound of "the blood / Come gargling from the froth-corrupted lungs."[33] In *Goodbye to All That*, Graves talks of the various noises of combat in ambivalent terms, almost as a kind of necessary evil. On the one hand, the bombardment of his sense of hearing is what eventually causes his own "neurasthenic twitching," yet on the other hand, his ability to distinguish threatening from unthreatening sounds is one of the keys to his survival:

> I find that my reactions to danger are extraordinarily quick; but everyone gets like that. We can sort out all the different explosions and disregard whichever don't concern us – such as the artillery duel, machine-gun fire at the next company to us, desultory rifle-fire. But we pick up at once the faint plop! of the mortar that sends off a sausage, or the muffled rifle noise when a grenade is fired.[34]

Noise thus acts both as psychic enemy and physical friend, and part of the strain of life at the Front is the contradictory need it instills in the soldier to both heighten and deaden his sense of hearing so as to be hyper-alert when awake yet able to fall asleep through cannon fire.

In an interview Graves gave in 1971, he would extend the poetic problem of indescribability beyond sight to include all the distinct noises unique to the Great War as well. "You can't communicate noise," Graves explained, "Noise never stopped for one moment – ever."[35] Among the War poets, the response to this aural dimension of incommunicability is prototypically modernist, in that it involves, at once, a falling back upon literary tradition and, simultaneously, a rejection of tradition in the search for newer, more vivid poetic forms. In *The Great War and Modern Memory*, Fussell details how the War poets drew heavily on what he calls the "Arcadian Resources" of the English pastoral tradition to create ironic contrasts between country life before the War and the muddy bleakness of life at the Front.[36] But to render the barrage of combat sounds, the War poets consistently draw on a different classical form, namely, the conventional vocabulary of the heroic epic. Homeric and Virgilian battle-words like din and clamor, clash and roar, rumble, bellow, and thunder are pervasive in any anthology of World War I poetry. Yet *Paradise Lost* is arguably an even more direct influence than the *Iliad* or *Aeneid*, and so much of the

War poet's diction for the noises of combat would seem to come from Milton's account of God's declaration of War against the legions in Hell:

> . . . . Peace is despaired
> For who can think submission? War then, War
> Open or understood must be resolved.
> He spake: and to confirm his words, out-flew
> Millions of flaming swords, drawn from the thighs
> Of mighty cherubim; the sudden blaze
> Far round illumined hell; highly they raged
> Against the Highest, and fierce with grasped arms
> Clashed on their sounding shields the din of war.[37]

Again in Book VI, in Raphael's account of the surprise attack by Satan's armies and the ensuing counterattack staged by the angels Michael and Gabriel, there is another war story which would have certainly resonated with any soldier on the Western Front:

> And clamor such as heard in Heaven till now
> Was never; arms on armor clashing brayed
> Horrible discord, and the madding wheels
> Of brazen chariots raged; dire was the noise
> Of conflict[38]

Echoes of Milton's "din of war" can be found in Owen, Graves, and Sassoon, all of whom use the word in their war poetry. In "The Sentry," Owen struggles to hear the voice of his blinded subaltern through the "dense din" of heavy artillery.[39] In "A Jealous Man," Graves writes of, "The thronged din of battle / Gaspings of the throat-snared / Snores of the battered dying."[40] Sassoon, in "Break of Day," writes of the soldier who "coughed and dozed, cursing the din" for troubling his attempt to rest.[41] Sassoon's most overtly Miltonic moment though comes in the poem "Counter-Attack," where one can easily detect the elevated diction from Book VI of *Paradise Lost* applied to the Great War with mock-epic grandeur:

> Mute in the clamour of shells he watched them burst
> Spouting dark earth and wire with gusts from hell,
> While posturing giants dissolved in drifts of smoke.[42]

While the War poets did reappropriate the elevated diction of classical War poetry, at the same time, they shared the general Modernist dissatisfaction with inherited poetic forms, albeit for graver reasons than those of an Ezra Pound or a James Joyce. The inadequacy of language to communicate the realities of the trenches therefore led them in the exact opposite direction as well, away from elevated diction and toward the incorporation of so-called lower dialects (e.g. Ivor Gurney's "The Silent One" or Owen's many dialect poems).[43] Going even "lower," so to speak, it also led them to one of the most primitive forms of language, that is, onomatopoeia. In many ways, onomatopoeia is an obvious solution to the problem of incommunicability. By virtue of the way it seamlessly overlaps sound and sense, semiotically speaking, it offers one of the most direct forms of language possible. As a result, the more grandiose battle-terms such as din and clamor are regularly paired within the same poem with simple and even silly imitations of common sounds—thuds and flops and booms and bangs. In Edmund Blunden's poem, "Two Voices," for example, "The howitzer with huge *ping-bang* / Racked the light hut" (emphasis added).[44] The speaker of Ivor Gurney's "The Silent One" tells us that he "kept flat, and watched the darkness, hearing bullets *whizzing* – / And thought of music" (emphasis added).[45] In Sassoon as well, all that din and clamor is rendered onomatopoeically, as the "*thudding* of the guns" or when "guns into mimic thunder burst and *boom*" (emphasis added).[46] Then finally, there is Wilfred Owen, who employed onomatopoeia arguably to greater effect than any other War poet, as we will see in more detail in the following section. In "The Last Laugh," his "Machine guns chuckled—Tut-tut! Tut-tut!"[47] Most relevant to this work, however, is the "stuttering rifles' rapid rattle" in his "Anthem for Doomed Youth," where the entire line mimics the rattling alliteratively, through its alternating /r/ and /t/ sounds.[48] Onomatopoeia stands therefore as one of the most significant ways in which the War poets broadened the poetic lexicon of their day. The effect in poems where elevated diction is juxtaposed with the various thuds and bangs is an ironizing of the noble purpose behind the War, a tragicomic sense of the pointless absurdity of trench warfare. Such devices also serve for the poets as a way of distancing themselves from more propagandistic forms of War poetry. Nothing plops or whizzes, in other words, in a poem like "Charge of the Light Brigade."[49]

In the following section, I will show how Wilfred Owen approaches these interrelated themes—noise, silence, and voice—through certain stylistic innovations related to his use of onomatopoeia. I will also show how Owen's corpus becomes organized around a series of questions related to problems of voice. Specifically, how does one hear, or speak, over the many clamors both literal (artillery fire) and metaphoric (the propagandizing of the press and the military) that drown out the more authentic voices of the War? How does one properly lend one's voice to the dead soldiers, the "millions of the mouthless dead" as the poet Charles Sorley calls them (or the "noiseless dead" in Sassoon's words), who cannot speak for themselves.[50] Prior to all of this, how does the War poet first restore their own voice, again literally, when suffering from war stammering (as in Owen's case) or metaphorically, how do they find a language capable of representing their traumatic memories?

"the new voice from Craiglockhart"

It is no exaggeration to state that Wilfred Owen's short period of intense poetic productivity (roughly August 1917–November 1918) was directly instigated by his being diagnosed with shell shock. Without that diagnosis, he would not have been transferred to the Craiglockhart War Hospital in Edinburgh, where he came under the care of Dr Arthur Brock, who encouraged the writing of poetry as a therapeutic exercise. He would have also missed out on the most formative moment of his brief poetic career, his meeting with fellow patient Siegfried Sassoon, who encouraged and critiqued Owen's first attempts at realistic war poetry. With respect to the debates about shell shock going on at the time, Owen's medical history represents a classic example of those ambiguous cases which sat, as Peter Leese puts it, on the "borderline of concussion and neurosis."[51] On patrol one night in March of 1917, Owen slipped and fell into a 15-foot cellar, hitting the back of his head on the way down. He tried to carry on but soon had to be taken to the 13th Casualty Clearing Station, where he was treated for symptoms of concussion. Back at the Front a few weeks later, Owen would undergo his most psychologically traumatic combat experience. During a reconnaissance mission, he and his men were pinned down and pummeled by German artillery for 12 straight days. When a shell finally hit the mark, Owen was blasted through the air into a nearby ditch. For the next several days, he took cover alongside the scattered body parts of his friend, Second Lieutenant Gaukroger. Having now undergone a second concussion in a matter of weeks, Owen was transferred back to the 13th Casualty Station, where he was able to update his mother on his health:

> Here again! The Doctor suddenly was moved to forbid me to go into action next time the Batallion goes. . . . I did not go sick or anything, but he is nervous about my nerves and sent me down yesterday – labelled Neurasthenia. . . . I still of course suffer from the headaches traceable to my concussion. Do not suppose I have had a "breakdown." I am simply avoiding one.[52]

It is easy to see how a case like Owen's would have straddled the border of neurogenic and psychogenic views at the time, with concussive and psychological forms of trauma happening to him concurrently. Initially, Owen understood the root cause of his neurasthenic symptoms in concussive terms, and it was only after he was treated by the prominent psychoanalyst Dr William Browne that he began to take a more psychogenic view of his situation. In a letter to his sister from 8 May 1917, his view on his neurasthenia shifts from talk of concussions to the effect of sharing the hole for several days with his dismembered fellow officer: "You know it was not the Bosche that worked me up, nor the explosives, but it was living so long by poor old Cock Robin (as we used to call 2/Lt. Gaukroger), who lay not only near by, but in various places around and about if you understand. I hope you don't."[53] Owen would spend several weeks at the Casualty Clearing Station, but when his neurasthenic symptoms showed no signs of improvement, he was transferred on 23 June 1917 to the ward of Craiglockhart War Hospital dedicated specifically to officers suffering from war neurosis. While the above letter shows that he spared his family little when it came to the horrors of the Front, he was unusually reticent when it came to his own symptoms. Apart from the occasional reference to "disastrous nightmares," headaches, or trench fever, Owen provides almost no information about his state. From Sassoon's account of the first visit paid to him by the awestruck younger poet, however, we know that in late August Owen still "spoke with a slight stammer, which was no unusual thing in that neurosis-pervaded hospital."[54]

At Craiglockhart, Owen was placed under the care of Dr Arthur Brock, the pioneer of the psychosocial treatment method known as ergotherapy. This approach shared the same compromised goal, with most other Wartime treatments for shell shock, of returning the soldier to a state of serviceability as expediently as possible. Brock's method for this focused on engaging the soldiers in various activities: public service, light work, hobbies, and so on. The theory behind Brock's working cure was that the shocks of War had turned his patients in on themselves, thereby detaching them from society at large to an unhealthy degree.[55] By putting his officers to work, Brock attempted to reinstill in them a sense of their continued role in public life. In Owen's case, noting the young man's artistic temperament, Brock recommended various literary assignments for his treatment. Brock also handed Owen the responsibility of editing the hospital's magazine, *The Hydra*, which he ran from July to his departure from Craiglockhart in November 1917. In his role as the self-described editor of "the new voice from Craiglockhart," Owen wrote satirical pieces poking fun at the public opinion of him and his fellow officers. In the issue from 1 September 1917, Owen even took on the taboo subject of malingering: "Many of us who came to the Hydra slightly ill are now getting dangerously well . . . . In this excellent Concentration Camp we are fast recovering from the shock of coming to England. For some of us were not a little wounded by the apparent indifference of the public and the press, not indeed to our precious selves, but to the unimagined durances of the fit fellow in the line."[56] Owen's reference to becoming "dangerously well" hints at the easy temptation for shell-shocked soldiers to malinger. Later in the same editorial, Owen broaches the topic more directly, in the style of a "Letters to the Editor" reply:

> One contributor seems so well in love with the life here that he writes inquiring:
>
>> Shall I mutter and stutter and wangle my ticket?
>> Or try another flutter and go back and stick it?[57]

In other words, the imagined soldier asks Owen in his role as editor, should I get my discharge home by faking a speech disorder or take the riskier bet, go back to the Front, and stick it out? Obviously, there is more than a little autobiography behind this. Whether or not to return to the Front was the question that weighed most heavily on both Owen and Sassoon during their stays at Craiglockhart. Like Sassoon, Owen felt as conflicted about being away from his soldiers as he did about leading them into death. In *The Poetry of Shell Shock*, Daniel Hipp explains how Brock's "working cure" would have exacerbated this moral quandary to officers like Owen: "he could resist the remedy and remain shell-shocked, incapable of doing anything or he could . . . prepare himself for the activity of bringing more suffering upon himself and others in the trenches."[58] To doctors like Brock, becoming well again meant an ethical return to work, but to the officers, returning to work meant leading more men into harm's way. It is easy to see, then, how malingering through the simple charade of a stutter would have offered a convenient and morally justifiable alternative to many officers. As Owen points out jokingly in the editorial, all he needed to do was perform his stammer a little longer to "wangle his ticket," that is, to obtain a medical discharge. In fact, however, we know from his letters that he asked Dr Brock the very same week he wrote this editorial about the date of his possible return to duty.

In his chapter "Wilfred Owen, Shell Shock, and Poetic Identity," Daniel Hipp argues that poetry offered a kind of third way out of Owen's moral quandary. He could maintain his shell-shocked status by muttering and stuttering, he could reassume his role as an officer, or he could go back to the Front in the role of a poetic witness. "Poetry," writes Hipp, "becomes for Owen the means to complete what Brock's methods had begun by enabling Owen to create a vision of his role as poet and spokesperson that would give his return to the trenches the moral purpose that the goals [sic] ergotherapy left out of the equation."[59] So what begins as therapy, putting his nightmares down on paper and gaining some mastery over them by molding them into poetic form, eventually leads to the higher *calling* of spokesperson for the soldiers who cannot speak for themselves. Surprisingly though, for Hipp, Owen's personal difficulties with speech would seem to play no role in his reflections on the vital importance of achieving a poetic voice. Rather, in Hipp's view, the possession of a stammer seems almost incompatible with poetic voice: "The stammer from which Owen suffered would soon leave, perhaps as soon as he began the process of developing a confident poetic voice."[60] This reference to confidence betrays the same view of the personality type of the stammerer which was beginning to emerge when Owen was writing. It implies that overcoming the stammer is the necessary precondition for the achieving of a fully poetic "voice," but in the context of Craiglockhart in 1917, the opposite would seem truer. Biographically speaking, Owen's development of his confident poetic voice did depend, after all, on the circumstances of his stammer placing him at Craiglockhart in the first place. Beyond that, the experience of the temporary loss of his own fluency, along with his living with dozens of other mute and stammering officers, certainly served more as inspiration than impediment in Owen's decision to dedicate himself to the writing of poetry. In short, his becoming a poetic spokesman depended as much (if not more) on his acquiring a stammer as on its overcoming.

Across Owen's corpus, these related issues lead him to thematize voice in myriad ways, and the word "voice" itself is used with a marked frequency, 15 times across his relatively small corpus. All voices, however, are not created equal for Owen, and there is a notable tendency toward the comparison and evaluation of the relative value of different voices in his poems. Predictably, the voice of the soldier is consistently privileged over the voice back home. His poem "Greater Love" offers the best example of the evaluative comparison of voices, in this case, between the speaker's two imagined loves. The voice of the beloved fellow soldiers is privileged over the voice of the beloved back home:

> Your voice sings not so soft, –
> Though even as wind murmuring through raftered loft, –
> Your dear voice is not dear,
> Gentle, and evening clear,
> As theirs whom none now hear,
> Now earth has stopped their piteous mouths that coughed[61]

Like Sassoon and others, Owen repeatedly haunts his poems with the ghostly half-muted voices of dead soldiers. In "Bugles Sang," the "dying tone / Of receding voices that will not return" is again compared with other voices, "Voices of old despondency resigned" and "Voices of boys . . . by the riverside."[62] The latter phrase is repeated verbatim in another poem, "Disabled," where the invalided veteran is depressed by the sound of children playing outside the hospital where he resides: "Through the park / Voices of boys rang saddening like a hymn, / Voices of play and pleasure after day."[63]

Owen's most systematic treatment of the interrelated themes of sounds and voice comes in a poem written 6 months after his return to the Front, "The Calls," a poem which also acts as his most definitive statement on the higher *calling* of the poet *qua* spokesman.[64] Each of the first five stanzas of "The Calls" is organized around a different type of sound: sirens, bells, organs, bugles, and gongs. What they are shown to have in common is their role of structuring quotidian time according to the different social institutions to which they correspond: labor, school, church, military discipline, etc. In her article, "Therapeutic Measures: *The Hydra* and Wilfred Owen at Craiglockhart War Hospital," Meredith Martin shows how metrical regularity in the poetic sense became tied up, in Owen's imagination, with the ergotherapy of Dr Brock, which stressed the importance of regularizing and disciplining one's time through work. Regarding "The Calls," Martin reads the poem as an allegory of sounds that is less satirical toward quotidian life than many of Owen's more canonical poems:

> Regularized external sounds, then, are allegorized in Owen's poems as a kind of suspicious discipline while, at the same time, the internal sounds of the poem ["The Calls"], contracting and expanding in his metrical manipulation, simultaneously support and reject this allegory. It is as if this earlier poem performs a kind of homage to the sounds and forms he makes ironic in "Dulce et Decorum Est" and other more directly critical war poems, whereas "The Calls" admits that the sounds and forms of military and literary discipline are necessary, but that Owen has no "proper" way to express this unfortunate necessity.[65]

Martin is certainly right that the attitude of "The Calls" is closer to homage than condemnation of the sounds of life back home. While he makes frequent use of his most comically effective device of onomatopoeia—the poem is full of moans, hums, buzzes, bumps and thumps, shrieks and sighs—they are certainly utilized less sardonically in this instance than in poems like "Dulce et Decorum Est," or "The Sentry," which I will analyze in more detail below. At the same time, what Martin reads as Owen's acceptance of the sound markers of quotidian life also acts to banalize them in the ears of the speaker. The model of the poet embodied in the speaker of "The Calls" is that of the lazy idle dreamer. Reminiscent of the speaker of Wordsworth's "The Tables Turned," rather than going to school when the bells chime, he lets Nature be his teacher, claiming simply, "I learn from the daisy."[66] He is likewise immune to the siren that tells the laborer it's time for work. Neither do the organs and amens of religion, nor even the military bugle move him to action. The new recruits may try to step in proper time, "But I sit still," he tells us, "I've done my drill." It is only the sound of suffering soldiers that compels him to action:

> Then sometimes late at night my window bumps
> From gunnery-practice, till my small heart thumps,
> And listens for the shell-shrieks and the crumps,
>   But that's not all.

> For leaning out last midnight on my sill
> I heard the sighs of men, that have no skill
> To speak of their distress, no, nor the will!
>   A voice I know. And this time I must go.[67]

Hence we find yet another instance of the privileging of the sounds of the Front, where the merest sigh of a soldier is valued higher than the "Stern bells" announcing the call to morning prayer. At the same time, however much empathy this poet-officer feels toward his subalterns in "The Calls," he still retains an elevated status over the "clumsy Tommies" he watches. In the final stanza, he occupies a literally elevated position, leaning out and listening from his sill, but he is also elevated through education (L. *educare*, to lift up) and temperament over the common soldier who is said to lack the skill and will to speak for himself. Wordsworth would seem relevant again for the model of the true Poet he articulates in the preface to *Lyrical Ballads*, as the one who speaks in the "real language of men" but is at the same time "distinguished from other men by a greater promptness to think and feel without immediate external excitement and a greater power in expressing such thoughts and feelings."[68]

These conflicted feelings of empathy and condescension toward his subalterns began, for Owen, long before his stay at Craiglockhart, at the intersection of class and language. In letters home, he regularly complained of the vile speech habits among the lower-class soldiers in his unit. Their every utterance, for him, formed part of the "universal pervasion of *Ugliness*. Hideous landscapes, vile noises, foul language and nothing but foul, even from one's own mouth (for all are devil ridden) . . ."[69] He even goes out of his way in one letter to compliment Sassoon on being "practically the only one in the place [Craiglockhart] who doesn't swear conversationally."[70] To his credit, Owen gradually learned to embrace this other "real language of men" and understand how linguistic phenomena like slang, nicknaming, and cursing were ultimately forms of play that helped the men build stronger bonds of camaraderie. Embracing the "vile language" of his underlings also meant incorporating lower-class dialects into his poems. His motivation for this might have had less to do with the overcoming of class barriers than with the poetic effect dialect offered, that is, yet another manner in which to render the sounds of the Front with more vivid directness. In any case, the result is the series of persona poems like "The Chances," written entirely in a Pygmalionesque dialect (with all aitches omitted) or "The Letter," in which the speaker switches between writing his own experience in his low-prestige dialect and speaking it to his fellow soldiers.[71] Needless to say, the sense of *speaking for* the common soldier is altogether different in these poems, and the lending of one's voice takes on a modernist sense of both impersonality and impersonation.

Unlike with dialect, the habit of cursing seems to have tested Owen's gentility too much for him to ever incorporate it directly. The closest he comes to recording the incessant swearing of his soldiers is in "The Last Laugh," which opens with the soldier's dying exclamation, "O Jesus Christ, I'm hit," but even there, the intent of the exclamation—"Whether he vainly cursed, or prayed indeed"—is left undecidable.[72] Nevertheless, as Daniel Hipp notes, Owen's attitude toward cursing changes quickly from his remarks about "vile language" in April–November 1917, when he admits in the poem "Apologia Pro Poemate Meo" to having "perceived much beauty / In the hoarse oaths that kept our courage straight."[73] It is worth noting here that Owen's firsthand experience of the fragility of language appears to have affected his thinking about voice in more ways than one, and his changed attitude on linguistic taboos likely had something to do with the experience at Craiglockhart of witnessing of his fellow officers struggle to regain fluency. In any case, cursing becomes a recurring theme in Owen's work, appearing in several other poems, including "The Sentry," "S.I.W.," "Music," "Sonnet," and the unfinished "Bugles Sang."[74]

The last two poems in this list offer an interesting contrast to the way noise and voice are approached in Owen's other war poems. In particular, both poems re-elevate the diction of battle and personify the noises of the guns as an act of *language*, specifically, as a curse which effectively drowns out the weaker voice of the common soldier. I have already noted several of the comedic sounds that guns make in Owen's poetry (guffawing, chuckling, etc.), but in "Sonnet: On seeing a piece of our artillery brought into action," the cursing of the guns is rendered instead as a highly poeticized magical incantation:

> Be slowly lifted up, thou long black arm,
> Great gun towering towards Heaven, about to curse;
> Sway steep against them, and for years rehearse
> Huge imprecations like a blasting charm!
> Reach at that Arrogance which needs thy harm,
> And beat it down before its sins grow worse;
> Spend our resentment, cannon, – yea, disburse
> Our gold in shapes of flame, our breaths in storm.

> Yet for men's sakes whom thy vast malison
> Must with innocent of enmity,
> Be not withdrawn, dark, thy spoilure done,
> Safe to the bosom of our prosperity.
> But when thy spell be cast complete and whole,
> May God curse thee, and cut thee from our soul![75]

With respect to the structure of arguments in this sonnet, it is well known that Owen generally preferred the English form over the Italian for the closing argument it allowed one to make in the rhyming couplet. Hipp also demonstrates that Owen regularly used the octave and sestet split to give voice to both the soldiers and those back home, allowing their viewpoints as thesis and antithesis to synthesize into the higher perspective of the poet. In this particular sonnet, Owen uses the convention of the volta, or turn of thought from octave to sestet, to sternly mark the separation between two types of soldiers: the one who is unabashedly grateful for his side's firepower versus the one who fights without giving in to a jingoistic hatred of the enemy.

The poem's many rarified words like "spoilure" and "imprecations," as well as the archaic thys and thous, all situate this sonnet in a more classical mode of War poetry. The tone can only be described as one of extreme solemnity, making it one of Owen's more nationalistic efforts, reminiscent of earlier drafts of "Anthem for Doomed Youth," before Sassoon edited it into a more neutral commentary on the evils of war. The solemnity of "Sonnet" derives mainly from the absence of Owen's characteristically ironic diction.[76] There are no thuds or bangs here. Even the "blast" in "blasting charm" is used figurally, a simile for the extremely abstract "imprecations" of cannon fire, rather than the more immediate sound effect one might expect. The central trope of heavy artillery as magical spell takes us back to Milton, or perhaps with Owen's usage of the Anglo-Norman archaism "malison," to another war writer who often wrote of charms and curses, Sir Thomas Malory. The Anglo-Norman form "malison" and the old French "maleicon" both derive from the Latin malediction, meaning a curse cast upon someone. In its most literal sense, though, a malison is simply an evil noise or bad sound. Through the etymology of "malison," therefore Owen manages to encapsulate all of the positive and negative valences attributed to noise and voice by Graves and the other War poets.

By troping the cannon's firing as a kind of speech act, a curse delivered against the enemy, Owen sets the cannon in the role of another voice competing against the more human voices of the soldiers. Owen's "Bugles Sang" is perhaps his most beautiful articulation of this battle of sorts that goes on between the machines that speak and the humans that cannot. Like every other poem we have examined thus far, it contains a litany of aural imagery, bugle hymns for the dead, voices of boys, resigned voices of the old, etc. Its conclusion, although unfinished, offers his most explicit articulation of the way that modern mechanized warfare drowns out the human voice:

[   ] dying tone
Of receding voices that will not return.
The wailing of the high far-traveling shells
And the deep cursing of the provoking [   ].

The monstrous anger of our taciturn guns.
The majesty of the insults of their mouths.[77]

One cannot help but wonder who (or what) would have fulfilled the act of "deep cursing" here. Although the elegiac tone of these two poems sets them far apart from most of Owen's more celebrated war poems, what they have in common is the frequent use of personification, specifically personification through speech, by making guns *speak* where human voices fail. I have already noted several of the human sounds that guns and cannons make in Owen's poetry. They guffaw and chuckle. They even stutter like the soldiers who pull their triggers. Evidently, these more comedic uses of onomatopoeia are also acts of personification, insofar as the sounds are human. By more traditional poetic standards, one could imagine John Ruskin chiding Owen for an abuse of what he termed "the pathetic fallacy." But Ruskin had only personifications of Nature in mind when he coined the term, and he faulted the poets who repeatedly endowed natural phenomena with human feelings (e.g. "cruel foam") for an excessive sentimentalism. No one could accuse Owen of that here, because the objects personified are consistently technological instruments of war. What we have instead is another example of what Fussell called the dichotomizing habit of the War poets. Owen's numerous talking machine-guns act as another ironic response to conventional Nature poetry, the representation of an antipastoral world in which the clamor of the machine effectively mutes the human.

With respect to the two poetic registers cited above—elevated battle terms and onomatopoeic sound effects—"The Sentry" is arguably Owen's most successful combination of these two modes to speak for his fellow soldiers.[78] One of the last poems he wrote before his death in November 1918, "The Sentry" represents the culmination of his short-lived mature style. The occasion for the poem was a particularly harrowing artillery bombardment in January 1917, in which Owen was pinned down in No-Man's Land for 50 hours and one of his servants was blinded by one of the blasts. As Owen explained to his mother at the time, he felt partly responsible for what happened to the sentry:

> In the Platoon to my left the sentries over the dug-out were blown to nothing. One of these poor fellows was my first servant whom I rejected. If I had kept him he would have lived, for servants don't do Sentry Duty. I kept my own sentries halfway down the stairs during the more terrific bombardment. In spite of those, one lad was blown down and, I am afraid, blinded.[79]

Because of this, Hipp considers "The Sentry" Owen's most direct confrontation of his combat experiences. Hipp also stresses the primarily therapeutic purpose behind writing the poem, since Owen was revisiting a traumatic event that clearly still haunted him almost 2 years after it took place. The poem is divided roughly into three sections (10, 17, and 10 lines long) of iambic pentameter with an incoherent rhyme scheme that jumbles tercets, quatrains, and couplets together (a-b-a, a-b-a-b, a-b-b-a, and a-a patterns are all present) to match the chaotic nature of the events described. The first section stages the scene of the speaker and his men trapped in "an old Boche dug-out" under heavy fire. Hipp points out how in this first section Owen treats the experience in terms of a "general bombardment of all their senses," emphasizing not only the sounds of "shell on frantic shell" but also the "smell of men" and the "slush waist-high" in which the men take cover.[80] The second section describes the blast that finally breaks through the dug-out and blinds the sentry. In this section, Owen's signature onomatopoetics takes over as noise again becomes the dominant form of sensory bombardment. The deprivation of sight in the blinding of the Sentry only draws greater attention to this emphasis on hearing. Despite the fact that Owen used the poem in part as a therapeutic tool to deal with his guilt over the fate of the soldier he rejected, his description of the blinding of the Sentry is rendered in a fashion that can only be described as comic:

> . . . . There we herded from the blast
> Of whizz-bangs, but one found our door at last, –
> Buffeting eyes and breath, snuffing the candles,
> And thud! flump! thud! down the steep steps came thumping
> And sploshing in the flood, deluging muck –
> The sentry's body[81]

The effect here is undeniably slapstick, with its rampant onomatopoeias, its exaggerated diction of thumping and sploshing, and the cartoonish use of exclamation points to emphasize each and every sound the sentry's body makes as it tumbles down the stairs. The use of exclamation points recalls Graves' similar construction in *Goodbye to All That*, in speaking of his dread of "the faint plop! of the mortar that sends off a sausage."[82] This unorthodox line could be parsed in many ways, but the most plausible metrical scanning would go as follows:

And **thud! flump! thud!** down the **steep steps** came **thump**ing

With the insertion of one 'foot' too many (or at least one syllable, depending on how one scans the line), Owen would seem to be punning metrically on the soldier's tripping down the stairs. The deliberately gauche ending of the line with a gerund, which closes the line on a weak unstressed syllable, further adds to the clumsy ridiculousness of the scene. The majority of gerunds in this section produce similar sound effects, from the "*thumping* and *sploshing*" of the sentry's body to the "*shrieking* air" with which the section ends (emphasis added). Finally, the sheer number of onomatopoeias should be underscored, not only the exclaimed thuds and flumps, but also the term for the specific artillery bombarding them. "Whizz-bang" was a nickname given by the British soldiers to the shells fired from the German 77-mm field gun, because the shell traveled faster than the speed of sound. Only the briefest *whizzing* sound was heard before the *bang*, giving soldiers almost no warning of its approach.

The overall effect of the second section could almost be called Chaplinesque, which is not that farfetched considering that Owen saw many of Chaplin's earliest films. We know that he enjoyed them enough to see some of them more than once, and he even made allusions to Chaplin in *The Hydra*, likening his physical antics to the state of the shell-shocked soldier. In the third and final section, however, Owen raises the tone from slapstick comedy to high tragedy. The speaker's memories shift to the gory aftermath of the battle, to "Those other wretches, how they bled and spewed," and his relation to the memory of these events is a simple desire for repression: "I try not to remember these things now." Not surprisingly, the diction of the final few lines elevates as well from onomatopoeic descriptions of the Sentry to the overtly Miltonic sounds of war that fail, for once, to drown out the soldier's voice:

Half listening to that sentry's *moans* and jumps,
And the wild *chattering* of his broken teeth,
Renewed most horribly whenever *crumps*
Pummelled the roof and slogged the air beneath –

Through the *dense din*, I say, we heard him shout
"I see your lights!" But ours had long died out. (emphasis added)[83]

The poet's ability here to empathize is severely compromised. Unlike the speaker of "The Calls," who is moved by the "sighs" of his men, this speaker admits to only "half listening" to the moans and chattering. They only add to the sensory overload of the moment, each time another shell hits the roof under which they cower with a loud *crumping* sound. As Hipp points out, however, the poet's role as spokesperson is preserved in spite of this by the simple insertion of "I say" into the penultimate line: "the phrase 'I say,' seems nothing more than a foot to fill out the line. However, this phrase provides Owen the opportunity to be the distinct poetic voice for all who have heard and seen himself included."[84] The exact noise over which the Sentry is heard, as I have already noted, is overtly Miltonic:

Through the ***dense din***, I **say**, we **heard** him **shout**

In what would seem to be further deference to Milton, Owen arranges the din into one of Milton's favorite forms, the spondee, and orders the line such that all the words to do with speaking and hearing receive stress.

In terms of a final statement by Owen on the complex thematic of voice and noise to do with the Great War, one could do much worse than requoting the above line: "Through the dense din, I say, we heard him shout." Any authentic speaking as poet for other soldiers, in this formulation, requires first a true listening, something which Owen admits in "The Sentry" posed its own challenges. The poet must find a way to hear over the shrieking curses of guns at the Front and the propagandistic voices back home, and to be heard himself, he requires a kind of poetry that doesn't just speak but shouts, in sound effects and exclamation points! These concerns were hardly unique to Owen, and Owen owes much to Sassoon, who thematized the antagonisms between voice, noise, and silence in equally interesting ways. One sees Owen's debt to his mentor most clearly in Sassoon's "A Whispered Tale," which compares yet another kind of noisy talk, the bragging of "fool-heroes" to the liminal, measured whispering of the shell-shocked soldier who feels no need to glorify his traumas. Of that ultimately wiser voice, Sassoon writes: "what you said /

Was like a message from the maimed and dead. But memory brought the voice I knew, whose note / Was muted when they shot you in the throat; And still you whisper of the war."[85] These lines help to remind us how the many metaphorical questions of voice that arise in the poetry of Owen, Sassoon, and others were always deeply rooted in their concrete experience of language breakdown. Both Owen and Sassoon witnessed the impact on their fellow soldiers of their speech disorders. For Owen, there is the added element of his personal experience of stammering. Only Sassoon would live to see the ongoing struggles these post-War stammerers faced.

Stuttering and Sexuality in Woolf, Melville, Kesey, and Mishima

"Ejaculation is at once a physiological and a linguistic concept. Impotence and speech-blocks, premature emission and stuttering, involuntary ejaculation and the word-river of dreams are phenomena whose interrelations seem to lead back to the central knot of our humanity."

– George Steiner, *After Babel*

"shy and stammering"

Immediately after World War I, the heightened social visibility of speech disorders like aphasia, war stammering and mutism began to manifest itself in popular cultural forms, and the increasingly commonplace association of stuttering with soldiering reached a saturation point where the condition was no longer linked specifically to the aftereffects of shell shock. One of the most popular songs from the period, "K-K-K-Katy," offers one such depiction of a soldier who stutters *prior* to heading off to War. Written in 1917 by the vaudevillian songwriter Geoffrey O'Hara, "K-K-K-Katy" was subtitled "The Sensational Stammering Song Success Sung by the Soldiers and Sailors."[1] The song tells the story of a soldier named Jimmy who falls in love at first sight with a maid named Katy during a military march:

Jimmy was a soldier brave and bold,
Katy was a maid with hair of gold,
Like an act of fate,
Kate was standing at the gate,
Watching all the boys on dress parade.

Jimmy with the girls was just a gawk,
Stuttered ev'ry time he tried to talk,
Still that night at eight,
He was there at Katy's gate,
Stuttering to her this love sick cry.

K-K-K-Katy, beautiful Katy,
You're the only g-g-g-girl that I adore;
When the m-m-m-moon shines,
Over the cowshed,
I'll be waiting at the k-k-k-kitchen door.

Since Jimmy's stutter is attributed simply to his shyness around girls, we see here one of the very first examples of the psychosexual model of the stuttering young man which began to emerge by the end of the War. This psychogenic paradigm of the nervous, sexually inhibited stutterer would become the dominant model for understanding such disorders for the next several decades. In the soldier Jimmy's case, when he finally does goes off to War, his stutter is rendered, again, not as a post-traumatic condition, but as an amorous comedy, part of the camaraderie of trench life for him and his fellow soldiers:

Now he's off to France the foe to meet.
Jimmy thought he'd like to take a chance,
See if he could make the Kaiser dance,
Stepping to a tune,
All about the silv'ry moon,
This is what they hear in far off France.

K-K-K-Katy, beautiful Katy,
You're the only g-g-g-girl that I adore;
When the m-m-m-moon shines,
Over the cowshed,
I'll be waiting at the k-k-k-kitchen door.

The connecting of stammering to the twitchy or shy soldier also becomes a staple in fictional portrayals after the War as well. In *Shell Shock*, Leese notes how, "in fiction the shell-shocked survivor quickly becomes a stock figure too, a sign of destroyed manhood back from the war and struggling to survive in the 1920s and 1930s."[2] The quintessential portrait of the shell-shocked veteran struggling to readjust to civilian life comes of course in Virginia's Woolf's *Mrs Dalloway* (1925). The character of Septimus Warren Smith is assumed by many critics to be loosely based on Siegfried Sassoon, because of the poetic sensibilities Septimus displays before the War in addition to their shared initials (S. S.) and eccentrically non-English Christian names. Woolf had taken an early interest in Sassoon because of his highly publicized statement of conscientious objection, "A Soldier's Declaration," and she would also write a review of his collection of war poems *Counterattack* in 1918. Many Woolf scholars also cite the study submitted to Parliament in 1922, *The Report of the War Office Committee of Enquiry into "Shell Shock,"* which publicly acknowledged that shell shock was an ongoing social issue, as a factor behind Woolf's relatively late decision to insert a shell-shocked character into *Mrs. Dalloway.*[3] In the two medical figures who treat Septimus, Doctor Holmes and Sir William Bradshaw, Woolf embodies the two competing views on shell shock laid out in the previous chapter, Holmes being a general physician and Bradshaw a psychiatric nerve specialist. Woolf is ultimately critical of both approaches, for too easily arriving at the conclusion that there is nothing actually wrong with a patient like Septimus. "Nerve sympoms and nothing more . . . there was nothing whatever the matter with him," Doctor Holmes informs Septimus' wife, Lucrezia.[4] Likewise, for Bradshaw, Septimus is just another nerve case, and the cure "was merely a question of rest."[5] It is only upon hearing of Septimus' suicide later that evening that Bradshaw and other members of the upper class are forced to reflect on "the deferred effects of shell shock" during Mrs Dalloway's dinner party.[6]

On the single day in which the novel takes place, in June 1923, Septimus is still presenting with hallucinations, tremors, and stammering. His most salient symptom, however, both clinically and metaphorically speaking, is his general state of desensitization. Septimus exhibits an inability to feel in the dual sense of a lack of sensation and of empathy. "He could not taste. He could not feel," he thinks to himself at one point, despite the fact that "his brain was perfect."[7] He also suffers from the guilt of being unable to feel affection from the touch of his wife or to feel anything about the death of his friend Evans in the War. Septimus' mild stammer surfaces during his rushed consultation with the psychiatrist Bradshaw:

"I—I—" he stammered.

But what was his crime? He could not remember it.

"Yes?" Sir William encouraged him. (But it was growing late.)

Love, trees, there is no crime-what was his message?

He could not remember it.

"I—I—" Septimus stammered.[8]

While many critics point to his stammer as a sign of his lingering shell shock, the fact that Septimus also stammers long before the War is a detail that is usually overlooked. The young Septimus, fancying himself a budding poet, runs away from his home in Stroud to London, where the barrage of new life experiences hardens him, changing his face, in a matter of 2 years, "from a pink innocent oval to a face lean, contracted, hostile."[9] To suggest the way the War cut short the potential of a whole generation of young men, Woolf poignantly condenses what might otherwise have been Septimus' *Bildungsroman* into a few simple lines. Employing a botanical metaphor, his experiences, she writes, "flowered from vanity, ambition, idealism, passion, loneliness, courage, laziness, the usual seeds, which all muddled up (in a room off the Euston Road) made him *shy, and stammering*, made him *anxious* to improve himself, made him fall in love with Miss Isabel Pole" (emphasis added).[10] Like the soldier Jimmy from the popular song, then, Septimus also stammers before he even volunteers for service, and it would seem for the very same reason, a shy nervousness around the woman he loves. The cause of Septimus' stutter, therefore, is less straightforward than being just another case of shell shock. The source of his overall pathology is partly environmental as well, in that the signs of nervousness to his personality are already present before the War, from the moment he moves to the big city. Woolf reminds us that, "London has swallowed up many millions of young men called Smith," and insofar as he embodies a common social type, Septimus is therefore reminiscent of Zola's "new individual" Laurent, whose bucolic temperament is rendered neurotic, or enervated by exposure to the many shocks (in the Benjaminian sense) of modern urban life.[11] In this sense, the stammer acts as the outward mark of an entire generation of twitchy, urban, postwar males.

The fact that Septimus already exhibits anxious stammering before he ever goes off to war is crucial for understanding how clinical views and cultural representations of the condition developed from the interwar decades through the post-World War II period. Woolf's decision to have Septimus stammer both before and after his war experience speaks to one of the most perplexing questions during the War with respect to shell shock. Members of the medical community struggled to understand why, for instance, when two soldiers witnessed an identical traumatic event, one soldier would develop acute shell shock while the other could continue to fight. Malingering was the most convenient explanation, but psychiatrists increasingly argued for predisposition. During treatment, they sought out signs of neurosis in the soldier's childhood in order to make a case for the relevance of the standard Freudian narrative of psychosexual development to the experience of War, or what Freud insisted was the peace-time ego's supervenience over the war-time ego.

Freud himself wrote relatively little about stuttering, and the historian Benson Bobrick in his book *Knotted Tongues: Stuttering in History and the Search for a Cure* has shown that it was not Freud himself but his disciples like Sandor Ferenczi, I. Peter Glauber, and Isador Coriat who did the conceptual work of mapping stuttering, in increasingly outlandish ways, onto the Freudian model of psychosexual development and the Oedipal complex.[12] In Ferenczi's most systematic response to Freud's views of human sexuality, *Thalassa: A Theory of Genitality* (1924), he connects stuttering and ejaculation to the processes of anal excretion and retention. While he admits that the ejaculation of semen is basically a urethric and excretory act, Ferenczi argues that the sex act itself is both urethric and sphincteric, both expulsive and retentive, insofar as the semen is withheld (for varying durations) and only released upon the overcoming of great pressure. Based on this, Ferenczi understands the opposite sexual problems of premature ejaculation and impotence in terms of the "unceasing struggle . . . between the evacuatory and the inhibitory, between expulsion and retension."[13] Impotence, from this vantage point, is caused by the "inhibitory influences" gaining an upper hand over the expulsory powers.[14] This leads Ferenczi to posit any and all problems of ejaculation as related forms of what he calls "genital stuttering."[15] For Ferenczi, as we see in the following citation from Chapter 1 of *Thalassa*, this link between stuttering and ejaculation is much more than mere analogy:

This assumption presupposes a highly complicated and finally graduated coordination, a disturbance of which would produce just that ataxia and dyspraxia which one may describe as premature and inhibited emission. One is thereby forcibly reminded of a certain similarity between the anomalies of seminal emission of which I have spoken and the speech disorder which goes under the name of stuttering. In this instance, likewise, the normal flow of speech is assured by the proper coordination of the innervations necessary to the production of vowels and consonants. But if speech is interfered with from time to time by impeded vocalization or by the spasmodic character of the enunciation of consonants, there result the varieties of stuttering which specialists in speech disorders refer to as vocalic and consonantal stuttering. It is not difficult to guess that I should like to compare the innervation necessary to the production of tone with urethrality, and the interruptions of tone by consonantal sounds, which are in many ways suggestive of sphincter action, with anal inhibition. Yet that this is no mere superficial parallel but on the contrary has reference to a fundamental similarity between the two pathological conditions which goes much deeper, is attested by the remarkable fact that the disturbances of innervation which characterize stuttering are in fact traceable psychoanalytically to anal erotic sources on the one hand and to urethral erotic on the other. In a word, I should like to conceive of the pathophysiological mechanism of disturbances of ejaculation as a kind of genital stuttering.[16]

In *Knotted Tongues*, Bobrick notes that these ideas probably stemmed from a passing remark Freud made in a letter to Ferenczi in 1915, where he suggested, "stuttering might have something to do with a conflict over excremental functions."[17] It is important to underscore here how literally Ferenczi takes this connection between genitality and stuttering, since we will shortly see how this connection is re-taken up and metaphorized in fiction. What we would today call erectile dysfunction is much more than *like* stuttering for Ferenczi, and likewise stuttering is much more than like sexual impotence, since the same underlying psychosexual mechanisms and tensions are at work behind both sets of phenomena.

The most influential psychoanalytic work on stuttering in the following decades stressed the importance of the relation to the mother as the determining factor in whether or not a child develops a stutter.[18] For Freudian speech pathologists like I. Peter Glauber and Isador H. Coriat, the psychopathology of the stuttering child always stems from an arrested development at the oral stage resulting in "an ego insufficiently differentiated from the mother."[19] In his 1943 article "The Psychoanalytic Conception of Stammering," Coriat goes so far as to suggest that the physical movements of the lips and tongue in the act of stuttering represent an unconscious reenactment of breast feeding: "In the speech of stammerers, the illusion or fantasy of nursing is maintained, and the original gratification is continued by this illusory substitution for the maternal nipple, the stammerer thus retaining his mother into adult life."[20] Based on this, Coriat further concludes that this "labile character trait" common to all stutterers determines the very sounds that they are most likely to find difficult to enunciate, the so-called *labial* consonants (*p*, *b*, and *m*), because the production of these particular sounds most closely approximates the act of sucking on the maternal breast.[21]

It should also be noted that the idea that stuttering was linked to certain personality types did not begin either with the Great War or with Freud. In *Knotted Tongues: Stuttering in History and the Search for a Cure*, Bobrick reminds us that as early as the mid-nineteenth century, "there were those who regarded stuttering as a personality disturbance or 'nervous disorder' of some sort."[22] In particular, Bobrick cites German theorists like Karl Ludwig Merkel and Reinhold Denhardt who understood and treated stuttering and other dysphonias as phobias. Much the way the condition of selective mutism is approached today in children, the stutter was thought to be caused by a "phonophobia," a fear of speech in which two volitionary forces existed in opposition to each other, in a sense canceling each other out. In the sections that follow, I will show how these two models gradually coalesce, first in Melville's *Billy Budd*, then in two portrayals of another generation of postwar males from Ken Kesey's *Cuckoo's Nest* and Yukio Mishima's *Temple of the Golden Pavilion*. Traces of the Freudian psychosexual account are already present in *Billy Budd*, intermingled with ideas of the stuttering young man as weak-willed. The three literary narratives I will examine in this chapter all contain elements of these two main psychogenic accounts of the personality type of the stutterer. The characters of Billy Budd, Billy Bibbit, and Mizoguchi are all portrayed as cripplingly timid, with a childlike or feminized form of weakness that prevents them from mastering their own tongue.

Relatedly, the stories of Billy Bibbit and Mizoguchi also reflect the dominant psychoanalytic conception of stuttering from this period, a view which I will show is already subtly prefigured in Herman Melville's *Billy Budd*. Kesey's mental patient and Mishima's Buddhist monk (and presumably Melville's foretopman as well) are virgins at the outset of their stories, and their sexual inexperience, as well as their stuttered speech, is troped together as interrelated forms of blockage. By contrast, the standard of fluent speech against which their stutters are measured is troped as the unblocked flow of words. While the linking of speech and sexuality has a history too long and complex to detail here, for this chapter, it suffices to point to the conceptual connection reflected in the etymology of the verb "to ejaculate," the senses of which include both the production of seminal fluid and the spontaneous or emphatic production of words. What distinguishes these three portraits of the stuttering male is the causal directness with which the associations between sexual ejaculation and fluent speech and between sexual repression and stuttering are made.

"organic hesitancy"

In his Introduction to *Cuckoo's Nest*, Robert Faggen calls attention to Kesey's indebtedness to various Melvillean characters, from the hints of Bartleby and Queequeg in Chief Bromden to the role of R. P. McMurphy as both Confidence Man and Captain Ahab for the other men on the ward. Regarding the two stuttering Billys, Faggen notes that "it's hard not to think of Melville's scapegoated Billy Budd in considering the fate of Billy Bibbit."[23] Before examining the portrayals of Mizoguchi and Billy Bibbit especially, it is necessary to revisit their most influential precursor, since Melville's novella anticipates virtually every twentieth-century stereotype about men who stutter. Billy Budd is at once infantilized and feminized, and though a fully developed man, he is said to look younger than he actually is, "owing to a lingering adolescent expression in the as yet smooth face all but feminine in its purity."[24] Fulfilling the sexually ambiguous role of the "Handsome Sailor," Billy is said to embody both a masculine ideal, making him an object of envy for the other men on board, and a refined beauty, which simultaneously marks him as a feminized object of homoerotic desire. In seeming contrast to his idealized status as the handsome sailor, Billy's "straightforward simplicity" also makes him, in the eyes of Melville's narrator, "little more than a sort of upright barbarian such perhaps as Adam presumably might have been ere the urbane Serpent wriggled himself into his company."[25] As critics like David Greven have noted, by describing Billy as a barbarian, Melville is obviously playing on the classical connotations of the term "barbarian," meaning originally one who stammers (from the Latin *balbus*) or a foreigner whose strange tongue cannot be understood (from the Greek *barbaros*).[26] At the same time, barbarism does not equal innocence, and so the further association of Billy with Adam before the Fall would seem also to idealize his straining for words, construing it not as the barbaric breakdown of fully formed language but rather as that first attempt at speech made by prelapsarian Adam in Genesis 2:19.

Billy Budd's actual stutter, while significantly less chronic than that of Billy Bibbit and Mizoguchi, still represents the most paradigmatic form of stuttering: the repetition of the initial consonant of the given word followed by schwa. Rare as his stuttering is, only occurring at moments of extreme agitation, Melville's graphic rendering of stuttered speech is even rarer. It happens only once in the entirety of the narrative, during the clandestine encounter in which Billy is approached by the afterguardsman and experiences what Eve Kosofsky Sedgwick has interpreted as a veiled form of homosexual panic.[27] In his eagerness to reject the afterguardsman's mutinous proposition, Billy's stutter "somewhat intruded: 'D–d–damme, I don't know what you are d–d–driving at, or what you mean, but you had better g–g–go where you belong! . . . . If you d–don't start I'll t–t–toss you back over the r–rail!'"[28] Despite his sudden panic, Billy's stutter is short-lived in this scene, only "somewhat" surfacing at the peak of his agitation. The moment the afterguardsman departs, Billy manages to "master the impediment" and is able to answer the forecastleman's inquiries into the incident.[29] Later on, when Lieutenant Claggart accuses Billy of mutiny, Billy experiences an even greater agitation in which his "lurking defect" devolves into a total blockage of the speech organs, producing not even a stutter but only "a strange dumb gesturing and gurgling . . . intensifying it into a convulsed tongue-tie."[30]

Earlier critics like Richard Chase and Charles Olson and more recent ones like Samuel Otter have all noted how Billy's "lurking defect" situates him alongside various other "maimed" characters throughout Melville's corpus, begging the question of whether speech disorders can be properly understood in the same terms as outwardly visible disabilities.[31] Of course, the well-known first description of Billy's "vocal infirmity" characterizes it in terms of an incongruence between a hidden defect and an outer perfection:

> Though our Handsome Sailor had as much of masculine beauty as one can expect anywhere to see; nevertheless . . . there was just one thing amiss in him. No visible blemish indeed . . . but an occasional liability to a vocal defect. Though in the hour of elemental uproar or peril he was everything that a sailor should be, yet under sudden provocation of strong heart-feeling his voice, otherwise singularly musical, as if expressive of the harmony within, was apt to develop an organic hesitancy, in fact more or less of a stutter or even worse.[32]

Melville's wording here leaves some ambiguity as to whether the amissness of this "one thing amiss" refers to the stutter itself or to some underlying moral or characterological defect of which the stutter is only a symptom. As the OED defines its primary adverbial sense, to be amiss means to perform something "erroneously, in a way that goes astray of, or misses its object."[33] Throughout the novella, the adjectival "amiss" acts as a recurring leitmotif for describing various types of indirection, both verbal and nonverbal, appearing six more times after its initial usage to describe physical or spiritual defects as well as more quotidian errors. When Billy finds himself in trouble below deck with one of the corporals, for instance, it is because there is "something amiss in his hammock," and in the naval chronicle's account of Billy's execution, it is reported that "nothing amiss is now apprehended aboard H. M. S. *Bellipotent*."[34]

But what does it mean exactly for language to be amiss? Unlike the more straightforward term for Billy's speech disorder, "organic hesitancy," which treats stuttering as an interruption of the organs of speech, the term "amissness" seems at first glance an unusual choice in that it would appear to conceptualize the stutter not as the absence or intermittence of fluency but rather as a kind of speech that misses its target. Insofar as the idea of amissness applies to Billy's stutter itself, there would seem then to be a blurring of any rigid distinction between standard fluent speech and stuttered speech, since Billy's verbal amissness is only one of many forms of indirect or amiss modes of speech that proliferate in the novella. Some of these strictly verbal amissnesses include the pith of the old Dansker, who like Billy is a man of "few words," as well as the act of false witness in the "sundry contumelious epithets" made by Claggart's underling, the corporal Squeak.[35] The narrator also attributes "equivocalness" to the "obscure suggestions" made by the afterguardsman to Billy.[36] The penchant for nicknaming among the sailors is yet another mode of indirect speech, in which the playful redundancy of a nickname is preferred to the indexicality of the proper name. Thus, Vere is also known as "Starry Vere," Billy as "Baby Budd," Claggart as "Jemmy Legs," and so on. Even Melville's narrator displays amissness in language when he suggests that describing Claggart's nature is "best done by indirection" or when he pauses awkwardly in Chapter 18 to justify his own use of analepsis, since "nothing especially germane to the story occurred until the events now about to be narrated."[37] Ultimately, Melville seems less interested in upholding some standard of fluency from which Billy's stutter could be said to fall short than in demonstrating the impossibility of any purely direct act of communication.

The notion of language as a metaphor for morality or character (in which fluent direct communication is a virtue and disordered or indirect speech a vice) is something Melville's own narrator again is clearly conscious of when in Chapter 4 he begs the reader's forgiveness for committing what he calls the "literary sin" of digression.[38] The most negatively charged portrayal of speech missing its mark appears of course with Claggart, whose "equivocal words" and "ironic inklings," as John Wenke has noted in his essay "Melville's Indirection," are a reflection of the "natural depravity" of his morals.[39] As an indirect two-sided kind of speaking in which one word can have many meanings, equivocation as a linguistic vice has traditionally been associated with the forked tongue of Satan, placing Claggart in the role of the "urbane Serpent" who tempts an innocent Adam. Contrary to the prelapsarian innocence of Billy's Adamic stammering, which never "[deals] in double meanings and insinuations of any sort," Claggart's equivocation therefore functions more like a willed speech disorder.[40] Yet if Claggart exists in strict moral opposition to Billy, when it comes to language, the polar opposite of Claggart's equivocation is not Billy's stutter but the univocal speech of Captain Vere, whose chief virtue of directness is to him crucial to maintaining order aboard the *Bellipotent*. Prior to the accusation scene, Vere is compelled to demand that Claggart be more direct when Claggart verbosely refers to Billy as a man who "had entered His Majesty's service under another form than enlistment."[41] Claggart's mistake in Vere's eyes is to employ the rhetorical device of circumlocution through this unnecessarily wordy description of Billy, when a much more succinct term, "impressed men," is available.[42] Yet even Vere's verbal directness has its limits, as we find at the moment Claggart makes an allusion (yet another indirect or amiss rhetorical device) to the Nore Mutiny. Vere quickly interrupts Claggart again, this time to insist on the need for tact, silence then being the only form of verbal indirectness ultimately sanctioned by Vere.

In the interactions between Claggart and Billy, these various moral connotations attached to speech are more directly tied to sexuality through Melville's etymological punning on the two senses of the word "ejaculation." First, Melville plays on both senses in the incident of the "streaming soup," when Billy trips and spills his soup in front of Claggart, who "was about to ejaculate something hasty at the sailor, but checked himself."[43] During the accusation scene, Melville keeps this twofold sense of ejaculation in play when Billy's inability to summon spontaneous speech leads to his eruption of violence toward Claggart. Unlike the other bluejackets who are able to "shoot at [Claggart] in private their raillery and wit," Billy has difficulty "shooting" his words when nervous, and so his arm shoots out instead: "The next instant, quick as the flame from a discharged cannon at night, his right arm shot out, and Claggart dropped to the deck."[44] The orgasmic overtones of this scene are completed when at last Claggart's "body fell over lengthwise, like a heavy plank tilted from erectness. A gasp or two, and he lay motionless."[45] What is most interesting here is that both the verbal and sexual connotations interact with each other in Billy's twofold "organic hesitancy" without the word "ejaculation" ever appearing in this particular scene. The glaring irony of course is that Billy's arm does what his speech organs cannot, namely, ejaculate in the primary sense of the term by "darting or shooting forth" (*OED*).[46] It is precisely because Billy's other organs are blocked that his only outlet is the physical (as opposed to verbal) form of striking out at Claggart. We know this is not the first time

Billy has substituted physical ejaculation for verbal, based on the report of an earlier incident aboard the *Rights of Man*, where Billy reacted to the threats of a fellow shipmate by "[letting] fly his arm" as "quick as lightening."[47] Even Billy himself is aware of the irony that he can only ejaculate in the primary sense, but not in the secondary sense with his tongue, when he explains to Vere in their final meeting, "Could I have used my tongue I would not have struck him. . . . I had to say something, and I could only say it with a blow."[48]

"m-m-m-m-mamma"

The name of Kesey's stuttering young man—Billy Bibbitt—serves not just as an overt onomastic reference back to his Melvillean precursor but also as an onomatopoeic play on his own difficulties with language. In other words, that Billy Bibbit's name itself performs a kind of stutter, a reduplication of the consonant-vowel cluster *bi-*, only strengthens the sense that Bibbit's identity can be reduced to his broken speech. Phonologically, Bibbit's stutter follows the same pattern as that of Billy Budd: the repetition of the onset syllable (consonant + schwa). Kesey's way of rendering Bibbit's stutter graphically varies, however, depending on the particular word being stuttered. While Melville leaves the schwa sound implied with a dash, Kesey chooses in most cases to inscribe a vowel (usually with an *e* or *uh*). For example, when Nurse Ratched inquires about Bibbit's difficulties with speech during one of the group therapy sessions, he informs the group that he "fuh-fuh-flunked out of college be-be-because I quit ROTC."[49] As might be expected, Bibbit's stutter coincides with moments of nervousness or shame, and its severity increases the more self-conscious or intimidated he becomes. When he is asked by Big Nurse to diagnose his own condition, Chief notices that he is "stuttering worse than ever because he's nervous" and is "choking on the word, like it's a bone in his throat."[50] Eventually, the severity of Bibbit's stutter reaches a sort of crescendo in the final confrontation with Nurse Ratched, when Big Nurse threatens to tell his mother about his first sexual encounter: "Duh-duh-don't t-tell, M-M-M-Miss Ratched. Duh-duh-duh—."[51]

As in Melville's novella, where the stutter is just one of the many things "amiss" with respect to language, so too the disturbances in Billy Bibbit's speech are only one of many forms of linguistic disturbance displayed throughout *Cuckoo's Nest*. There are the incoherent outbursts of Old Pete Bancini, "who opened and closed his mouth to talk but he couldn't sort the words into sentences any more," not to mention Ruckly's favorite copralalic utterance, "Ffffuck da wife."[52] The speech of the Swedish sailor Rub-a-dub George is both accented and mumbled because he always talks with his hand pressed to his mouth until somebody "pulled the hand away so's the words could get out."[53] Among the staff as well, there is the psychoanalytic jargon (or psychobabble) of Doctor Spivey's "Therapeutic Community" as well as the indirect accusations behind the "calm schoolteacher tone" of Nurse Ratched, who, much like Claggart, is said to have "a genius for insinuation."[54] Most importantly, there is the heavily colloquial style of Chief's narration which marks him, like Billy, as someone partially estranged from the apparatus of standard fluent English owing to Chief's dual ethnic background as the son of a white mother and an Indian father. Chief's narration is littered with folksy contractions and grammatical errors rooted in an oral understanding of English, for example, when he says of the black boys, "they should of knew better'n to group up and mumble together."[55]

Of course, Chief's estranged relation to standard fluent English goes well beyond the folksiness of his narration and comes closest to Billy Bibbit's through his feigned mutism. It is this mutism, along with his feigned deafness, that provides Chief with the anonymity and access required to act as the semiomniscient narrator of the goings-on around the ward. Chief's voluntary form of speech disorder, if we can call it that, was triggered by a traumatic childhood experience in which three white appraisers visited his father's lands with plans to convert the tribal waterfalls into a hydroelectric dam. The strangers mock the young Bromden's skin tone and one of them calls him "little Hiawatha" because they assume he cannot possibly speak English.[56] When the young Chief tries to shame them with what he calls his "very best schoolbook language," he is surprised to find "the apparatus inside them take the words I just said and try to fit the words in here and there, this place and that, and when they find the words don't have any place ready-made where they'll fit, the machinery disposes of the words like they weren't even spoken."[57] What Chief is describing here is obviously not literal but cultural deafness. The counterpoint to this scene comes during another moment of linguistic disturbance, when Chief struggles to understand the comically nonsensical propositions of Colonel Matterson. Occurring between Billy's accounts of the origin of his stutter and of his flubbed attempt at a marriage proposal, this interlude between the Colonel and Chief suggests a more organic model of language as an instrument of empathy:

> His voice as deep and slow and patient, and I see the words come out dark and heavy over his brittle lips when he reads.
>
> "Now . . . . The flag is . . . . Ah-mer-ica. America is . . . the plum. The peach. The wah-ter-mel-on. America is . . . the gumdrop. The pumpkin seed. America is . . . tell-ah-vision."
>
> It's true. It's all wrote down on that yellow hand. I can read it along with him myself.
>
> "Now . . . . The cross is . . . . Mex-i-co." He looks up to see if I'm paying attention, and when he sees I am he smiles at me and goes on. "Mexico is . . . the wal-nut. The hazelnut. The ay-corn. Mexico is . . . the rain-bow. The rain-bow is . . . wooden. Mexico is . . . woo-den."
>
> I can see what he's driving at. He's been saying this sort of thing for the whole six years he's been here, but I never paid him any mind, figured he was no more than a talking statue, a thing made out of bone and arthritis, rambling on and on with these goofy definitions of his that didn't make a lick of sense. Now, at last, I see what he's saying. I'm trying to hold him for one last look to remember him, and that's what makes me look hard enough to understand. He pauses and peers up at me again to make sure I'm getting it, and I want to yell out to him. Yes, I see. Mexico is like the walnut; it's brown and hard and you feel it with your eye and it feels like the walnut. You're making sense, old man, a sense of your own. You're not crazy the way they think. Yes . . . . I see . . ."
>
> But the fog's clogged my throat to where I can't make a sound.[58]

In the previous scene, the appraisers fail to process the Chief's words, not because of what he is saying, but because of who he is. His message is heard but discarded, despite being put in his "very best schoolbook language." But in Chief's encounter with Colonel Matterson, the terms are reversed.

The breakdown in communication stems not from who Matterson is, but from what he's saying. Matterson's "lessons," as Chief calls them, recall the particular kind of nonsense language outlined by Noam Chomsky in *Syntactic Structures*. Chomsky famously demonstrated the difference between syntax and semantics by crafting the grammatically correct yet theoretically meaningless sentence: "colorless green ideas sleep furiously."[59] Without the mutually contradictory qualifiers of Chomsky's example (green and colorless), Matterson's sentences offer an even more streamlined proof of the same argument. Propositions like "America is the plum" and "Mexico is the walnut" represent the most basic building blocks of linguistic meaning, the "S is P" statement. Yet by virtue of their meaningless content, they also suggest the possibility of an endlessly reproducible form of nonsense language. Despite the semantic obstacle, along with the Colonel's painfully slow mode of delivery, a degree of mutual understanding is still achieved because the Chief remains open to the possibility that the Colonel might say something worth hearing. Chief is therefore able to access the extraliteral sense behind the Colonel's lessons (Mexico is *like* a walnut), whereas the appraisers remained unable to process even the literal. This inability or unwillingness on the part of the whites to process the words of a young Indian boy reminds us that the apparatus of standard fluent language, as a machine, is no less prone to breaking down than the rusty organs that produce Billy's stutters and Chief's silences. Quite the contrary, for Kesey, the machine-like apparatus of standard English exhibits its own forms of breakdown all the time.

The link first established in *Billy Budd* between repressed sexuality and stuttered speech is made much more simplistic, even reductive, in *Cuckoo's Nest*. For Billy Bibbit, the blockage of his sexual organs does not merely coincide or correlate with the blockage of his speech organs. Rather, his prolonged virginity is shown to be the primary cause of his stutter and his loss of virginity its instantaneous cure. Although Billy Bibbit does not exhibit any of Billy Budd's feminine or homoerotic qualities, Kesey does carry Melville's stereotype of the infantilized stutterer over into his portrayal of Billy Bibbit. Chief notes of the 31-year-old Bibbit that "in spite of him having wrinkles in his face and specks of gray in his hair, he still looked like a kid—like a jug-eared and freckled-faced and buck-toothed kid."[60] This infantilization that prolongs

Billy's virginity (along with his stutter) takes on clear Oedipal overtones through the domineering influence of his mother. Mrs Bibbit is a receptionist in the lobby of the hospital where her son resides and a neighbor and friend of Nurse Ratched as well. In Chief's description of her, she is "a solid well-packed lady with hair revolving from blond to blue to black and back to blond again every few months."[61] Her relationship with Billy corresponds almost too neatly to the model of the jealous mother developed by Freud in his *Three Essays on the Theory of Sexuality*. As Freud famously wrote: "A man especially looks for someone who can represent his picture of his mother, as it has dominated his mind from his earliest childhood; and accordingly, if his mother is still alive, she may well resent this new version of herself and meet her with hostility."[62] This possibility of shifting the Oedipal conflict—in which the rivalry is not between father and son for the affection of the mother, but between mother and younger woman for the love of the son—was one of the factors that for Freud reduced the likelihood of young men resolving their Oedipal complex in any completely healthy way. Mrs Bibbit's status as a stereotypical Freudian mother is revealed when Chief recalls a disturbing incident during one of her visits:

> Billy's mother took the opportunity to leave her work and come out from behind the desk and take her boy by the hand and lead him outside to sit near where I was on the grass. . . . Billy lay beside her and put his head in her lap and let her tease at his ear with a dandelion fluff. Billy was talking about looking for a wife and going to college someday. His mother tickled him with the fluff and laughed at such foolishness.
>
> "Sweetheart, you still have scads of time for things like that. Your whole life is ahead of you."
>
> "Mother, I'm th-th-thirty-one years old!"
>
> She laughed and twiddled his ear with the weed. "*Sweet*heart, do I look like the mother of a middle-aged man?"
>
> She wrinkled her nose and opened her lips at him and made a kind of wet kissing sound in the air with her tongue, and I had to admit that she didn't look like a mother of any kind.[63]

Kesey leaves us with little room for doubt that any potentially therapeutic value to living on the ward is nullified by Mrs Bibbit's constant access to Billy. It is further nullified by the presence of the Big Nurse, who acts as a second mother to him, periodically reinforcing his sense of maternal guilt. "Good Morning, Billy," Ratched tells him, "I saw your mother on the way in and she told me to be sure to tell you she thought of you all the time and knew you wouldn't disappoint her."[64] Similarly, when Billy mentions a botched marriage proposal he once made to an unnamed girl, Nurse Ratched is there to reimpose his mother's jealousy as well: "Your mother has spoken to me about this girl, Billy. Apparently, she is quite a bit beneath you."[65] Here Kesey rehearses what was by that point a stock scene in portrayals of stuttering young men—the stuttered proposal—which along with the stuttered response to roll call, is rehashed time and time again in popular cultural forms for its blend of pathos and comic relief. Another song from the same era as "K-K-K-Katy," titled "Oh Helen," features a lovesick stutterer named Willie Meet who "tho' good at grammar / When he'd speak, he'd always stammer."[66] William's lovesick overtures get him into trouble with Helen's father when his stutters are mistaken for a series of fetishistic profanities:

Oh H-H-Hel
Oh H-H-Hel
Oh Helen please be mine
Your f-f-feat
Your f-f-feat
Your features are divine
I s-s-swear
I s-s-swear
I swear I will be true
Oh D-D-Dam
Oh D-D-Dam
Oh Damsel I love you

It bears pointing out that the diminutive Willie, short for William, is often interchangeable with Bill or Billy. Another well-known song from the post-War era, "You Tell Her I Stutter" (1922), features yet another stuttering Billy who finds a different solution to the problem of proposing:

Bill McCloskey was a husky, healthy handsome lad;
And McCloskey had a pretty little girl by the name of Pear

But McCloskey, big and husky, stuttered very bad
So when he wanted her to marry him
He told her brother Jim
You, you, you, you, you, you tell her
Cause I, I, I, I, I stutter..[67]

In his cultural history *Stutter*, Marc Shell dates this lighthearted tradition of stuttering songs back to an eighteenth-century ballad, "Goody Groaner: The Celebrated Stammering Glee."[68] Shell delineates three types of verbal substitution used as coping strategies by stutterers. The first of these, interlinguistic synonymy, is an act of bilingualism where a synonym from another language is substituted for the word the speaker struggles to enunciate. The second strategy, intralinguistic synonymy, which is frequently employed in *Looney Tunes* by Porky Pig, involves the substitution of a synonym from the same language. The story of Bill Mccloskey offers an example of the third form, what Shell calls personal substitution, where the stutterer seeks out a surrogate to speak on his behalf.[69] As Shell points out, this puts the stutterer in the degrading (or in the case of a marriage proposal, emasculating) position of a ventriloquist's dummy. With respect to masculinity, Bill McCloskey and the Jimmy from the song "K-K-K-Katy" deviate from the more strictly neurotic model of the stutterer in that they are depicted as physically strong. The pathos of their situations derives therefore from them being healthy young men who, like Billy Budd, tragically have just "one thing amiss" about them. When Pearl consents to marry Bill Mccloskey through his ventriloquist, Bill instantly thinks ahead to the vows he will have to make:

When, when, when I hear the parson say,
Will you hon, hon, honor and obey?
I'm afraid that I will answer
Eepp-eipp Gimmee a piece of peipp

McCloskey thus indicates a fourth possible form of substitution—written for verbal (which we will return to in the following chapter in our study of Robert Graves' *I, Claudius*)—when he plans on asking for a piece of paper to write out his vows. Part of the comedy of this verse comes from Mccloskey transplanting his stutter onto the imagined Parson, raising the uncomfortable question of whether a ceremony where the questions were stuttered and the answers were written down would be legally binding. It seems no accident that all of these songs and cartoons relate to situations and utterances that qualify in J. L. Austin's terms as speech acts: pledges, vows, proposals, and so on.[70] It is likewise no accident that when asked to speak on the subject of his own stutter, Billy Bibbitt focuses on two situations that depend on something not unlike Austin's illocutionary force: asking "will you marry me?" and saying "I'm here." The humiliation of struggling to assert his mere presence, by saying "here," leads Billy to drop out of ROTC. Subsequently, he becomes prone to the same feelings of invisibility that haunt the Chief.

In terms of how this relates to Bibbit's sexuality, the implication that Billy's stutter forms part of an unresolved Oedipal complex is made even more explicit when he is asked to recall the first word he ever stuttered: "Fir-first stutter? First stutter? The first word I said I st-stut-tered: m-m-m-m-mamma."[71] Not surprisingly, in the Oedipalized case of Billy Bibbit, there is no mention made of Mr Bibbit, and it is only when McMurphy supplants Nurse Ratched as a father figure that Billy's sexual organs and organs of speech are simultaneously unblocked. McMurphy's mastery over his own voice is one of the many indicators, along with his calloused hands and unselfconscious laughter, that he is in full possession of his masculinity. His voice is described as "clear and strong, slapping up against the cement and steel," and his laughter likewise "spreads in rings bigger and bigger til it's lapping against the walls all over the ward."[72] Just as Chief's mutism persists until McMurphy is able to help him grow "bigger," so too Billy Bibbit is only able to overcome his stutter when McMurphy pushes him to lose his virginity.[73] Anxious during the lead-up to this rite of passage with the prostitute Candy, Billy says, "Look, McM-M-M-Murphy, wait!" McMurphy replies, "Don't you mamamamurphy me, Billy Boy. It's too late to back out now."[74] The pun in Kesey's alternate spellings suggests that even R. P. himself by this point understands Billy's pathology in quasi-Oedipal terms. That prolonged virginity was the direct cause of Bibbit's version of organic hesitancy becomes undeniable the morning after Billy sleeps with Candy, when, for the first and only time in the novel, Billy speaks with unimpeded fluency:

"Good morning, Miss Ratched," Billy said, not even making any move to get up and button his pajamas. He took the girl's hand in his and grinned. "This is Candy."

The nurse's tongue clucked in her bony throat. "Oh, Billy Billy Billy—I'm so ashamed for you. . . . What worries me Billy" she said, I could hear the change in her voice, "is how your poor mother is going to take this."[75]

Not only are there no traces of a stutter in this brief exchange, but the stutter seems to have been displaced momentarily onto Nurse Ratched. The bone that was originally stuck in Billy's throat, as he tried to articulate his own condition, now becomes the "bony throat" of Nurse Ratched. It is in this light as well that one should read both Billy's method of suicide (slitting his own throat) and McMurphy's subsequent decision to choke the Big Nurse. Choking Nurse Ratched suggests more than just a silencing of the ward's matriarch and a symbolic restoration of the traditional gender hierarchy. It is also an imposing of Billy's stutter onto her so that she experiences the feeling of choking on one's words.

Earlier in the novel, when Chief eavesdrops on the group therapy session in which Billy's stutter is discussed, Chief notes dismissively that the group is "talking some nonsense about Billy's stutter and how it came about."[76] While Chief listens, "the words get dim and loud, off and on," almost as though one form of nonsense (the technical jargon of psychoanalysis) was being used to explain another (the incoherence of stuttered speech). Later on, when McMurphy questions Harding about the weakness endemic to the men, Harding answers, "Oh, I could give you the Freudian reasons with fancy talk and that would be right as far as it went. But what you want are the reasons for the reasons and I'm not able to give you those."[77] Considering Kesey's well-known skepticism regarding psychoanalytic talk and psychiatric practices like electroshock therapy, it should come as some surprise, then, that his portrayal of the root cause of Billy's stutter would fall back on the most basic of psychoanalytic theories. After all, while the term "psychobabble" would not be coined until 1975, 10 years after the publication of *Cuckoo's Nest*, Kesey's satire of psychiatric practices and psychoanalytic jargon largely fostered the notion that 1940s- and '50s-style Freudianism was a pretentious and meaningless form of nonsense masquerading as knowledge. Nonetheless, what Kesey ultimately gives us in the etiology of Billy's stutter are Freudian reasons without the fancy talk.

So why would Kesey revert to such an overdetermined Oedipal model of the stuttering young man? One possibility has to do with what most critics consider Kesey's misogynist views of the detrimental effects changing gender roles had on the post-World War II American male. Ironically, it seems that the misogynist approach to gender roles that underlies Billy's stutter resituates *Cuckoo's Nest* in the very tradition it set out to critique, that is, the socially conservative Freudianism first popularized in America in the 1940s through works like Edward Strecker's *Their Mothers' Sons* (1946) and Philip Wylie's bestseller *Generation of Vipers* (1942).[78] For Wylie as for Kesey, the so-called crisis of masculinity after World War II stemmed directly from the crippling influence of the American mom on that particular generation of young men. In *Generation of Vipers*, Wylie applies a similarly Oedipal framework of psychosexual development almost prescriptively to American society, coining the term "momism" to account for the American male's excessive attachment to his mother and the mother's overprotectiveness of her son. Consequently, the parallels between Mrs Bibbit and the Wyliean mom are so strong that portions of Wylie's *Generations of Vipers* read almost as if they were written with Billy's mother in mind: "Her policy of protection . . . was not love of her boy but of herself, and as she found returns coming in from the disoriented young boy in smiles, pats, presents, praise, kisses, and all manner of childish representations of the real business, she moved on to possession."[79] Kesey's portrayal of Nurse Ratched as Billy Bibbit's second mother also closely mirrors Wylie's language for describing the American mom as "a middle-aged puffin with an eye like a hawk that has just seen a rabbit twitch far below."[80] Billy and the other men think of themselves in exactly the same Wyliean terms as "feeble, stunted, weak rabbits," whose masculinities have been compromised by the wolves of the "juggernaut of modern matriarchy."[81] McMurphy echoes Wylie's condemnation of the "rapacity of loving mothers" when he boasts to the men that Nurse Ratched "fooled [him] with that kindly little old mother bit for maybe three minutes . . . but no longer."[82] Given Kesey's views on the fractured masculinity of the postwar American male, it is somewhat less surprising, then, that Billy Bibbit's speech disorder would be framed in

Freudian terms, where the sexual repression of "momism" is thought to create an entire generation of weak young men for which the stutterer stands as its primary symbol.

"the rusty key"

Based on the burning of Kyoto's Kinkakuji (Golden Temple) in 1950 by the Buddhist priest Hayashi Yoken, *Kinkaku-ji* [*The Temple of the Golden Pavilion*] acts in part as a commentary on what Yukio Mishima perceived to be the similarly fractured masculinity characteristic of postwar Japan. According to newspaper accounts, Hayashi had in fact been afflicted with a stutter from childhood, one of the few details from Hayashi's life that Mishima borrows in his invention of Mizoguchi as an awkward and introspective acolyte in training for the priesthood. Mizoguchi is unlike Billy Budd and Billy Bibbit in one crucial respect, however, in that he is the narrator of his own story. Although he never represents his own stutter graphically, he does render stuttered speech once in the novel in a scene where his stutter is mimicked by a fellow classmate and Mizoguchi chooses to inscribe this act of ventriloquism into the text: "I'm a st-st-stutterer" [*Do-do-domori nan desu*].[83]

Instead of Billy Budd's feminized beauty, Mizoguchi tells us he possesses a "conventional sort of ugliness" due to his "frail, ugly body."[84] Initially, he understands his speech disorder in conventional terms as a function of his generally weak constitution, suggesting the model of the weak-willed stutterer whose frailty prevents him from mastering his own tongue:

> I had suffered since my birth from a stutter, and this made me still more retiring in my manner. . . . My stuttering, I need hardly say, placed an obstacle between me and the outside world. It is the first sound that I have trouble in uttering. This first sound is like a key to the door that separates my inner world from the world outside, and I have never known that key to turn smoothly in its lock. Most people, thanks to their easy command of words, can keep this door between the inner world and the outer world wide open, so that the air passes freely between the two; but for me this has been quite impossible. Thick rust has gathered on the key.[85]

This sense of the blockage of speech as an obstacle dividing one's inner self from the outer world is underscored by the pun contained in Mizoguchi's own name. As David Pollack points out in his article on the novel, "Mizoguchi means literally 'estrangement-mouth' or 'rift-mouth.' It is his stuttering mouth, 'that silly little dark hole,' that creates an alienating and unbridgeable 'gulf' between him and the world."[86] In this regard, Mizoguchi's stutter poses obvious difficulties to his advancement as a Zen Buddhist, acting as an existential stumbling block in his attempts to achieve enlightenment. Throughout the novel, Mizoguchi associates the "slight delay" of his stutter with the overall disjointedness that prevents him from being able to unify his inner self with the outer world.[87]

Though the source of his stutter is never asserted quite as definitively as it is with Billy Bibbit, Mishima also turns to the figure of the dominant mother to account for Mizoguchi's pathology. From an early age, Mizoguchi saw his father grow increasingly frail from tuberculosis, and the formative moment of Mizoguchi's childhood came when he witnessed his mother having sex with one of her own relatives, even though her son and her dying husband were sleeping in the very same room. This traumatic experience was intensified by the fact that Mizoguchi's father lay awake the whole time, covering his son's eyes. In her article "A Manifestation of Modernity: The Split Gaze and the Oedipalised Space of *The Temple of the Golden Pavilion*," Rio Otomo points out the fundamentally gendered dichotomy resulting from this primal scene, whereby "the mother represents corporeality, ignorance, and profanation, while the Father represents spirituality, knowledge, and sacredness."[88] Otomo, however, glosses over the topic of Mizoguchi's stutter, and so any connection between his stutter and what she calls the "Oedipal conditioning" of his relationship with his mother is left unexplored.[89] At the same time, the received idea about the detrimental effects of domineering mothers on stuttering males has become such a commonplace that the jacket copy of the 2001 Vintage edition of *Golden Pavilion* can matter-of-factly state about this traumatic scene that "because of the boyhood trauma of seeing his mother make love to another man in the presence of his dying father, Mizoguchi becomes a hopeless stutterer."[90] While the mother's violation of the father's masculinity certainly plays a primary role in Mizoguchi's pathology, the causal relation between his speech disorder and this childhood trauma is hardly as straightforward as the jacket copy suggests, considering that Mizoguchi reports having suffered virtually since birth from a stutter and does not witness his mother's infidelity until the age of 13. Nevertheless, the role of maternal guilt in his dual blockage (sexual and vocal) resurfaces when his mother visits him at the Golden Temple shortly after his father's death:

> "The only thing for you now is to become the superior of the Golden Temple here [. . . .] You understand, dear? That's all your mother will be living for now." [. . . .] My "fond mother" had put her mouth directly against my ear when she was speaking to me and now the smell of her perspiration hovered before my nostrils [. . . .] Distant memories of being nursed, memories of a swarthy breast—the images raced unpleasantly round my brain. In the flames of the lowly field fires there existed some sort of physical force and it was this that seemed to frighten me [. . . .] "Yes," I answered, stuttering violently, "but for all I know, I'll be called up and killed in battle."
>
> "You fool!" she said. "If they start taking stutterers like you in the army, Japan is really finished!"
>
> I sat there tensely, filled with hatred for my mother.[91]

One finds here virtually the same imposition of maternal guilt as with Mrs Bibbit, as well as the same mildly incestuous interactions between mother and son, and while Mizoguchi may differ from Bibbit in his more active hatred of his mother, he is ultimately no more able to counteract her dominance. The fact that the memory of his mother's breast is followed immediately by a moment of violent stuttering lends itself to exactly the kind of Oedipal reading put forward by Coriat, where the fixation on the act of breast-feeding is unconsciously manifested through the stutter.

As in the cases of Billy Budd and Billy Bibbit, Mizoguchi's blocked speech is also repeatedly linked to his prolonged virginity: "Just as when some important words were trying to break free from my mouth and were blocked by my stuttering, this impulse was held burning in my throat. This impulse was a sudden desire for release."[92] Mizoguchi does not lose his virginity until late in the novel, and only after he is pushed to have sex by Kashiwagi, a fellow student at the Otani University whose loud laughter recalls the role played by R. P. McMurphy in Billy Bibbit's life. Kashiwagi walks with a pronounced limp due to having two clubfeet, and Mizoguchi is initially drawn to Kashiwagi through their shared experience of disability. Kashiwagi urges him to embrace his stutter, even to exploit it, as Kashiwagi does with his own clubfeet, so as to elicit pity from women. This only leads to a series of failed sexual encounters, for instance, when Mizoguchi is seated beside a flower arrangement teacher and feels paralyzed before the woman's naked breast. When he finally overcomes his feeling of impotence and sleeps with the prostitute Mariko, the unblocking of his sexual organ does result in the unblocking of his speech organs as well: "The law of distance that regulated my world had been destroyed . . . . After I had taken off my clothes, many more layers were taken off me—my stuttering was taken off and also my ugliness."[93] The fact that his stutter returns the very next day, however, suggests that the loss of virginity is never more than a temporary cure.

The sexual impotence that torments Mizoguchi throughout most of the novel resolves in the climax into a more basic frustration over his general lack of willpower. From the outset, Mizoguchi has not understood his speech disorder as the symptom of a more fundamental inability to act but, on the contrary, has understood his inability to act as a symptom of the overabsorption in words brought on by his stutter: "When action was needed, I was always absorbed in words; for words proceeded with such difficulty from my mouth that I was intent on them and forgot all about action."[94] The idea that words inhibit action is arguably the most autobiographical aspect of the novel for Mishima. In his memoir *Sun and Steel*, Mishima notes that from a very early age, words and actions existed for him in a "willfully created antinomy."[95] After Japan's defeat in 1945, the classicist Mishima sought to dissolve this antinomy by "reviving the old Japanese ideal of a combination of letters and the martial arts, of art and action."[96] In the case of Mizoguchi, this antinomy between words and actions eventually takes the form of an internal struggle over whether or not to set fire to the Golden Temple.

The desire to burn the temple is hardly the first time Mizoguchi understands action in purely destructive terms. In several scenes, he exhibits an impulse to destroy or deface beautiful things, such as when in middle school he takes the sword of a naval hero and makes several "ugly cuts" on its ornate scabbard.[97] The defacing of the sword is the first of many "small desecrations" that culminate in the burning down of the Golden Temple.[98] His relationship to the beauty of the temple follows the same isolating pattern as his stutter inasmuch as its beauty is said to cut him off from life, worsening his impotence by rendering him incapable of action. As a result, he comes to see its beauty as the true repressive force responsible for his stutter: "The suspicion had just crossed my mind that it might be my very conception of beauty that had given birth to my stuttering."[99] Since his stuttered words are an impediment to action, he believes that willing himself to act by burning the temple will offer a permanent cure. Moments before setting fire to the temple, he is therefore convinced that, "the rusty key that opened the door between the outer world and my inner world would turn smoothly in its lock. My world would be ventilated as the breeze blew freely between it and the outer world."[100] For Mishima himself, the ultimate goal of dissolving his "willfully created antinomy" was not destruction but a form of artistic creation that overcomes the sterility of art by unifying words and actions through the body. But in the case of Mizoguchi, his repression remains too severe for him to ever resolve the antinomy of words and actions through means other than destruction.[101]

Stuttering, Violence, and the Politics of Voice in Robert Graves, Philip Roth, and Gail Jones

"Feminas verba balba decent"

– Horace

"vox populi"

The popular model of democratic political agency, understood in terms of making one's voice heard, can be traced back to the Roman expression *vox populi*, the voice of the people, an expression which implies that political power resides in openly expressed public opinion. While the advocates of every type of identity politics have adopted this vocal metaphor at one point or another, the more fundamental issue of fluency is rarely raised in discussions of political marginalization. From the vantage point of this study, however, it is easy to see how fluent speech itself can become politicized, as a measure of one's relative empowerment, and how the figure of the stutterer, the aphasic, or the mute might stand (as it did for the World War I poets) for the one whose views cannot be heard in the public sphere.[1]

On the other side of this political coin, History is somewhat surprisingly full of politicians, lawgivers, orators, and monarchs who stutter. The best-known example of the stuttering leader is, of course, Moses, the vehicle of divine law who provides his people with the commandments by which they should live. Due to his troubles with speech, Moses must call upon Aaron to be his interpreter and spokesman when it comes to leading his people to freedom. This seemingly oxymoronic figure of the stuttering leader can be found in numerous other cultures as well. It is well known that the Greek orator Demosthenes suffered from a speech impediment as a child and allegedly overcame it by declaiming with pebbles in his mouth so as to strengthen his articulation. In sixteenth-century Native American history, the Iroquois lawgiver Dekanawida, because of his stutter, relied much like Moses on his spokesman Hiawatha to help him unify his tribes into the Iriquois Confederacy. In the fight for Irish independence, the figure of Charles Stewart Parnell stands out as yet another politician who rallied his people in spite of his severe difficulties with speech. This "Irish Moses," as James Joyce once referred to him, suffered from a stammer which he never overcame, but which did not stop him from leading the Irish people in the Home Rule movement of the 1880s.[2] One final example (recently popularized in the film *The King's Speech*) is the case of Prince Albert, who reluctantly took the throne as King George VI in 1936, after his brother's sudden and scandalous abdication. Albert's reluctance to become King stemmed largely from the lifelong stammer which made his many public-speaking duties a difficult and oftentimes humiliating burden.

"though he do limp and stammer a bit"

Only 2 years before George VI ascended the throne, almost prophetically, Robert Graves completed the first of his two historical novels about the Roman Emperor Tiberius Claudius Caesar Augustus Germanicus who, much like George VI, assumed the monarchy with great reluctance following a period of turmoil. The parallels between King George VI and the Emperor Claudius become almost uncanny when one considers their virtually identical physical impairments. Both monarchs suffered from childhood not only from a stutter, but also from similarly chronic stomach ailments as well as infirmities of the leg that left them with a noticeably limping gait. In literary history, the closest corollary to Claudius is arguably Mishima's stuttering monk. Like Mizoguchi, Claudius narrates his own story, although from the outset, as I will discuss further below, Claudius is at pains to reassure the reader of the reliability and authenticity of his authorial voice. Claudius also seems to share Mizoguchi's reluctance to transcribe his own disordered speech. Early in the first volume, when Claudius reports his visit to the Sibyl to seek a prophecy, he renders his stammer with ellipses: "'O Sib . . . Sib . . . Sib . . . Sib . . . Sib . . .' I began. She opened her eyes, frowned and mimicked me: 'O Clau . . . Clau . . . Clau . . . .'"[3] The more silent and temporal use of ellipses here suggests the strict distinction between stammering, or the prolonged inability to produce sounds, and the repetition of syllables (usually onset syllables) that comes with stuttering. Apart from this early visit to the Sibyl, Claudius almost never transcribes his speech disorder directly again, choosing instead to allude to its occurrence and then summarize what he was trying to say.

Claudius also shares with Mizoguchi the same weak constitution that marks his broken speech as the outward sign of an inner defect. Speaking of his older brother Germanicus and his older sister Livilla, Claudius notes, "both inherited my father's magnificent constitution. I did not. I nearly died on three occasions before my second year."[4] His young body is said to be "a very battleground of diseases," where conditions like malaria, measles, erysipelas, colitis, and infantile paralysis debate over "which should have the honour of carrying me off."[5] There is little consensus among medical historians about the root cause of the actual Claudius' various infirmities. Many, beginning with his own mother, believed that his symptoms were due to his premature birth. Others, including Claudius himself, understood his overall symptomatology as the consequence of polio, or as he describes it, "infantile paralysis which shortened my left leg so that I was condemned to a permanent limp."[6] From an early age, Claudius also presented with a variety of ticcish symptoms, which along with his stutter, led his family to believe he was impaired as much mentally as physically. In Graves' account, Claudius understands his many tics as an internalized fear over the disapproval of his parents and the threat of punishment for his embarrassing behavior: "The nervous tic of my hands, the nervous jerking of my head, my stammer, my queasy digestion, my constant dribbling at the mouth, were principally due to the terrors to which, in the name of discipline, I was subjected."[7] Recently, medical historians have suggested Tourette's syndrome as another possible explanation for his motor tics, and since tourettic movements and tourettic speech can sometimes be mistaken for a jerky stammering, his speech disorder might have formed part of this neurological syndrome which was entirely misunderstood in Antiquity.

Finally, Claudius also shares the fact of a troubled upbringing with characters like Mizoguchi and Billy Bibbit, though this part of his autobiography is related to us without the Freudian/Oedipal overtones we find in the latter cases. His father Drusus dies when Claudius is only an infant. Once a young man, Claudius seeks to fill this paternal void by asking anyone who knew Drusus, whether "senator, soldier, or slave," what his father was like.[8] Relatedly, the first work of history he attempts is a biography of his father, but the project is aborted when his grandparents deem the republican ideals expressed in it potentially treasonous. In addition to the absence of a strong father figure (a virtually universal feature of stuttering narratives, as we have seen), Claudius also suffers as a child from painful relations with his mother and grandmother. In this case, however, the mother issues are more a matter of neglect than of the Wyliean overprotective doting we saw with Billy Bibbitt: "It will be supposed that my mother Antonia . . . would have taken the most loving care of me, her youngest child, and even made a particular favorite of me in pity for my misfortunes. But such was not the case. She did all that could be expected of her as a duty, but no more. She did not love me."[9] Preferring her healthy and heroic firstborn Germanicus, Antonia considers her sickly child a "human portent" of bad events to come and even hints it would have been wiser to leave Claudius exposed on a hillside in the manner of the Greeks.[10] "Since I was an affectionate child," Claudius admits, "my mother's attitude caused me much misery."[11] Thus, we find in Graves' narrative a slightly revised model of the familial factors at work in the development of the stuttering personality type, constrained in certain ways by the source material and the dictates of the historical novel. It goes without saying that an overtly Freudian reading would be anachronistic in a first-person historical novel set during the Roman Empire, but Graves' self-described puritanism, as well as the historical Claudius' own prudishness (compared to the debaucheries of Tiberius and Caligula), seems to factor in to the general downplaying of psychosexual issues in both volumes of the autobiography. When he first falls in love as a teenager, Claudius exhibits at most a slight sexual shyness, and it is only his beloved Camilla who attributes his stammer to a nervousness around girls. "But I stammer. My tongue's a Claudian too," jokes Claudius, to which Camilla replies, "Perhaps that's just nervousness. You don't know many girls do you?"[12] While Claudius' experiences of being a husband are a source of comedy and humiliation throughout both volumes—his first marriage is to the tall lesbian Urgulanilla and he is later cuckolded by his final bride, the beautiful nymphomaniac Messalina who sleeps with virtually every man in Rome—there are no suggestions of prolonged virginity or sexual impotence, again largely dictated in this case by the source material.

During this period, conditions like stammering were treated largely as problems of elocution, and so it falls to Claudius' tutors to help him overcome his difficulties with speaking. His first tutor, Cato the Censor, takes a severe disciplinary approach to Claudius' many mistakes during recitation: "every time I stumbled over a word I used to get two blows; one on my left ear for stupidity, and one on my right for insulting the noble Cato."[13] The results are predictably poor. It is only when Athenodorus takes over for Cato that Claudius begins to show improvement in public speaking along with the signs of an intelligence far above the idiocy his family assumes of him:

> Athenodorus never beat me and used the greatest patience. He used to encourage me by saying that my lameness should be a spur to my intelligence. Vulcan, the God of all clever craftsmen, was lame too. As for my stammer, Demosthenes the noblest orator of all time had been born with a stammer, but had corrected it by patience and concentration. Demosthenes had used the very method that he was now teaching me. For Athenodorus made me declaim with my mouth full of pebbles: in trying to overcome the obstruction of the pebbles I forgot about the stammer and then the pebbles were removed one at a time until none remained, and I found to my surprise that I could speak as well as anyone. But only in declamations. In ordinary conversation I still stammered badly.[14]

Clearly then, the question of cause is much less fraught in *I, Claudius* than in works like *Cuckoo's Nest* or *Temple of the Golden Pavilion*, and there is likewise no epiphantic moment of total cure (whether sexual or destructive) as in the works of Kesey and Mishima. Rather, his stammer remains a gradual matter of setbacks and progress, humiliating public recitations and unexpected moments of eloquence where a quickness of wit (and of tongue) saves his life. The issue of the improvement of his stammer is further complicated by the dangerous political times in which he finds himself, during the reigns of Augustus,

Tiberius, and Caligula, when political rivalries spelled the assassination of several members of his family, including his grandfather, his uncle, his father, and his brother Germanicus. It has been suggested that Claudius deliberately exaggerated his physical and vocal infirmities to be perceived as a harmless fool, particularly to his grandmother Livia and his nephew Caligula. In *I, Claudius*, Graves has the historian Pollio suggest this feint to Claudius, during that formative scene where Claudius debates the merits of different styles of historical writing with Pollio and Livy. While Livy is off looking for a book, Pollio discreetly asks the young Claudian if he wishes to live a long life. When Claudius replies that he does, Pollio advises: "Then exaggerate your limp, stammer deliberately, sham sickness frequently, let your wits wander, jerk your head and twitch with your hands on all public or semi-public occasions. If you could see as much as I can see, you would know that this was your only hope of safety and eventual glory."[15] Again, there is historical evidence to support this theory. Many contemporaries of the actual Claudius noticed the sudden improvements to his limp, as well as his speech, very shortly after he was chosen to succeed Caligula. In this respect, Claudius is ultimately closer to a Chief Bromden than a Billy Bibbitt, feigning infirmity to avoid the notice of the dangerous powers that surround him. Late in life, when the Greek physician Xenophon is hired to be Claudius' personal physician, he even admits that he would prefer not to be better: "I assured him it was not only too late to do anything about my infirmities, but that I had grown quite attached to them as an integral part of myself, and that I had no use for Greek doctors."[16] Claudius finds a cagey, defensive kind of strength in his physical and vocal disabilities, something we will see again in the case of Merry Levov from *American Pastoral*. As a result, through his role as a historian, Claudius' attention shifts from overcoming his personal stammer to overcoming the instabilities and infelicities inherent to language itself via the clarity of historical writing.

It is Athenodorus who first instills in Claudius a sense of the value of disciplined clarity both in writing and in speech: "He first applied this discipline to my writing, then to my declamations, and finally to my general conversation with him . . . he never let any careless, irrelevant, or inexact phrase of mine pass without comment."[17] With respect to the practice of History, Athenodorus also emphasizes a clarity of presentation which eventually places Claudius in the camp of Pollio, whose plainer style is presented as the polar opposite of the more florid and dramatic style of Livy. As a result of Athenodorus' tutelage, Claudius comes to abhor many of the same "vices" of language I located in the previous chapter in *Billy Budd*, forms of ambiguity, redundancy, and indirectness such as circumlocution, nicknaming, and narratorial digression. *I, Claudius* opens with a diatribe against the many nicknames he has assumed over the years: "I. Tiberius Claudius Drusus Nero Germanicus. This-that-and-the-other (for I shall not trouble you with all my titles) who was once, and not so long ago either, known to my friends and relatives and associates as 'Claudius the Idiot,' or 'That Claudius,' or 'Claudius the Stammerer,' or 'Clau-Clau-Claudius.'"[18] While his motives in this instance are more hurt feelings than linguistic prescriptivism, Claudius revisits the problem of the ambiguity and redundancy of Roman names a few pages later:

> In compiling my histories of Etruria and Carthage I have spent more angry hours than I care to recall puzzling out . . . whether a man named So-and-so was really So-and-so or whether he was a son or grandson or great grandson or no relation at all. I intend to spare my successors this sort of irritation. Thus, for example, of the several characters in the present history who have the name of Drusus—my father; myself; a son of mine; my first cousin; my nephew—each will be plainly distinguished.[19]

Beyond the questions of naming it deals with, the entire first chapter of *I, Claudius* acts as a kind of narratorial apologia, where Claudius reassures the reader of the reliability and clarity of the story to follow. Moreover, in the second chapter, in place of a muse of divine authority, Claudius offers up the Sibyl's prophecy as further evidence of the authority of his text. Above all though, Claudius stresses the importance of a direct and chronological presentation of facts, with somewhat ironic effect, since these meta-discussions on the writing of history usually represent his most long-winded digressions. Of the ordering of his work, Claudius tells the reader that, "like all Roman histories this is written from 'egg to apple': I prefer the thorough Roman method, which misses nothing, to that of Homer and the Greeks generally, who love to jump into the middle of things."[20] Similar to Melville's narrator, he also begs the reader's forgiveness for the linguistic vice of digression at various points, for instance, when he veers from the story of a predicament faced by his brother

Germanicus, making "a very ill-judged digression" about the poor reception his satirical book *How to Win at Dice* had received.[21]

All of his linguistic prescriptions, along with his general contempt for eloquence, do ultimately relate for him back to the personal issue of his stammer. By privileging plain, direct speech over false eloquence, Claudius believes he has found a long-term solution to his basic difficulties with communication, a solution that will leave him fluent in the eyes of posterity while the texts of his contemporaries are all left stammering. This solution is the fourth kind of verbal substitution discussed in the previous chapter, namely, the substitution of the written word for the spoken: "when all other authors of to-day whose works survive will seem to shuffle and stammer, since they have written only for to-day, and guardedly, my story will speak out clearly and boldly."[22] Ironically, Claudius draws this conclusion based on his interpretation of the most ambiguous and opaque of texts, the prophecy of the Sibyl, whom he visits 18 years before the writing of his autobiography:

> Ten years, fifty days and three,
> Clau—Clau—Clau—shall given be
> A gift that all desire but he.
>
> To a fawning fellowship
> He shall stammer, cluck and trip,
> Dribbling always with his lip.
>
> But when he's dumb and no more here,
> Nineteen hundred years or near,
> Clau—Clau-Claudius shall speak clear.[23]

The dumbness mentioned in the final stanza implies that final "mutism" of death. The Sibyl thus reminds Claudius that we are all mute in the end, and it is only through the posthumous "fluency" offered by the written text that he will eventually "speak clear." While his general attitude on language is undoubtedly prescriptivist, Claudius does show here an openness to interpretation and a respect for poetic and prophetic forms of ambiguity that goes against his general views on "the proper presentation of facts."[24]

His less rigidly prescriptivist side is most apparent in the changes he proposes to the Latin language. The three new letters that were proposed by the historical Claudius raise an interesting question about how much of Claudius' views on language should be attributed to Graves himself, whose poetry is notoriously antimodernist in its stubborn clarity, and how much can be said to reflect the views of the actual Claudius.[25] The three letters Claudius proposed, which were officially inserted into the Latin alphabet, but fell out of use after his assassination, correspond to the modern letters /W/ and /Y/, and the Greek double-consonant Psi. Claudius also proposed that dots be placed between words, going against the convention of *scripta continua*, where no demarcation or separation was made from one word to the next.

His stated motive behind this linguistic reform is to make Latin "truly phonetic," but his method of implementing the change, once Emperor, is interestingly democratic.[26] Rather than simply decree his new letters be made part of Latin henceforth, Claudius puts the matter to a plebiscite and argues his case on the grounds of the inevitability of linguistic change: "I pointed out that though one was brought up to regard the alphabet as a series no less sacred and unalterable than the year of months, or the order of the numerals, or the signs of the Zodiac, this was not really so: everything in this world was subject to change and improvement."[27] It is here that we begin to see how language itself becomes politicized in the Claudius novels and how the figure of the stammerer serves as a symbol in modern fiction for the struggle to achieve (and in Claudius' situation, hold onto) political voice. For Claudius, letting the future state of the Latin language be a democratic matter stems not only from a personal sensitivity over his own "truly phonetic" difficulties, but also from his republican ideals, particularly with respect to the issue of free speech.

When it comes to his own account of his reign as Emperor, Graves' Claudius is best described as an unreliable narrator, maintaining the pretense of the objective historian, and operating in the classical mode of apologia to justify the events that led to him being made Emperor, his acceptance of the position only under fear of death, his many acts of imperial authority, and finally, his constant need to postpone the restoration of the Republic for which he spends the entire first volume arguing. His sudden rise to power, which occurs hastily in a matter of two pages at the conclusion of *I, Claudius*, is a clumsy unplanned act of mob rule, furthering his characterization of himself as a kind of plainspoken everyman, in spite of his obscure academic interests.

The nomination is made by one of the very same sergeants who capture him during the chaos that ensues after Caligula's assassination: "What's wrong with old Claudius for Emperor? The best man for the job in Rome, though he do limp and stammer a bit."[28] This farcical nomination is seconded and confirmed by the other assembled soldiers: "Loud cheers, laughter, and cries of 'Long live the Emperor Claudius!'"[29]

After the initial period of stabilization, still finding that the time is never quite right to restore the Republic, Claudius' compromise is to focus his efforts on restoring freedom of speech to Rome. Evidently, the exercise of "free speech" is an act overladen with symbolism and paradox in the tale of a stammering and democratically inclined, though sometimes tyrannical, Emperor. In Roth's *American Pastoral* as well, we will see how the very idea of free speech becomes a kind of double-entendre with respect to the marginalized stutterer who seeks to assert their voice in politics. The reforms that Claudius enacts take various civic and legal forms. He repeals the law instituted by Tiberius making certain forms of slanderous speech akin to treason. Following his military victory over the Britons, he also encourages the carnivalesque custom of allowing soldiers to mock their leaders, and "the veterans exercised their right of free speech which was theirs for the day, indulging in sarcastic ribaldry at the Victor's expense."[30] The night after his triumphal return, Claudius even disguises himself to mingle among the common people and hear their real thoughts on his military capacities, expressing the Voltairean sentiment, "I was glad that free speech had returned to Rome at last, after its long suppression by Tiberius and Caligula, even though some of the things I heard did not altogether please me."[31]

His most significant acts toward restoring free speech, however, involve his many reforms of the legal system. Perhaps partly out of envy, from an early age, Claudius feels a strong contempt for orators and the rhetorical tricks of their trade. As Emperor, he takes an especially active role in the courts, applying the preferences for clarity and succinctness which he learns from Athenodorus to the Roman judicial process. He admits a bias to rule in favor of orators who present their case in a brief and lucid way, and he works to remove the weight of eloquence from the scales of justice, both for the defendants and for their representatives. "I encouraged the appearance of a new sort of advocate," he writes, "men without either eloquence or great legal expertness, but with common sense, clear voices and a talent for reducing cases to their simplest elements."[32] The most controversial reform which Claudius introduces is the one for the defendants themselves:

> . . . my extraordinary decision in insisting that every man who appeared before me in court should give the usual preliminary account of his parentage, connexions, marriage, career, financial condition, present occupation, and so on—*with his own mouth, as best he could*, instead of calling upon some patron or lawyer to do it for him. My reasons for this decision should have been obvious: one learns more about a man from ten words which he speaks himself on his own behalf than from a ten-hour eulogy by a friend. It does not matter so much what he says in those ten words: what really counts is the way in which he says them. (emphasis added)[33]

There is a tension here between Claudius' dogmatic views on the value of plainspokenness, on the one hand, and his personal desire as someone who stammers, on the other hand, to create a space in which every man can speak for himself, "with his own mouth," however fluently or dysfluently. This act of identity politics on his part backfires because the public sees it more as a compulsion to explain oneself than as an expansion of their right to speak on their own behalf. Claudius is surprised to find that the public prefers the verbal substitution of counsel over the opportunity to defend themselves with their own mouths.[34]

Historians like Tacitus and Suetonius have tended to characterize Claudius as an inept ruler, rather than the appeasing and even deferential Emperor he makes himself out to be in *Claudius the God*, though his reputation in recent years has been rehabilitated by some. Whether Claudius' republican belief in free speech and his goal of restoring the Republic were genuine, it cannot be doubted that he also exhibited a tyrant's taste for violence throughout his 13-year reign. His exuberance for gladiatorial combat is often noted. His temper was so volatile at times that he even made a public apology for it while he was Emperor, and he had no qualms about executing dozens of senators and other conspirators as well as his adulterous wife, Messalina, along with several of her more regular consorts. For these reasons, the figure of Claudius, both historically and in Graves' fictionalization, represents a fascinating mixture of the self-effacing stutterer and the bloodthirsty despot. Any causal link one might try to find between the two tendencies, however, can only be said to remain below the surface in the Claudius novels. But this causal link continues to be a part of modern fictional portrayals in increasingly explicit forms, beginning as we have seen with Melville, continuing with Yukio Mishima and resumed, as we will see below, by the contemporary novelists Philip Roth and Gail Jones.

"angry because she stutters"

With Philip Roth's *American Pastoral* and Gail Jones' *Sorry*, we now turn our attention to how portrayals of the condition of stuttering, along with the stuttering personality type, are expanded in contemporary fiction to include implications for young women. As noted above, this particular speech disorder is significantly less common in women. The ratio of adult male stutterers to female stutterers is anywhere from 3 to 1 to as high as 5 to 1 in some studies, a discrepancy that continues to perplex researchers in the field of speech pathology.[35] In literary narratives about stuttering, the meaning attached to this speech-fluency disorder varies according to gender, reflecting diametrically opposed gender norms with respect to fluent, copious speech. The several portrayals of men we have examined to this point (from Billy Budd to Billy Bibbit) adhere to popular psychogenic conceptions of the personality type of the stutterer as either too weak-willed or nervous to assert himself through speech. By contrast, portrayals of women who stutter respond to a very different and conflicting set of expectations: for women to be both silent and articulate at the same time. Thus, for men, the stutter can be said to act as an internal trope of self-repression and represents a failure to live up to gender expectations. For women, the stutter acts instead as an external trope for social repression, representing a refusal of gender expectations.

In Philip Roth's *American Pastoral* (1997) and Gail Jones' *Sorry* (2007), the portrayals of stuttering in the female characters Merry Levov and Perdita Keene share the other common conception of the stutterer as someone who is prone to violent, destructive behavior. The characters of Merry Levov and Perdita Keene are both precociously intelligent, well-behaved, and seemingly incapable of aggression. Yet both girls commit extreme acts of violence while still at a young age: 16-year-old Merry bombs the local post office and 10-year-old Perdita stabs her father to death. Although the manifestations of their stutters are different—Merry develops hers gradually, whereas Perdita's stutter is triggered by the trauma of killing her father—both narratives share this same tendency to link blocked speech to sudden outbursts of violence. For both novels, as we will see, the association of violence and stuttering is further tied to the sense of political agency understood in terms of voice. This takes the form in Merry's case of her stuttering protests against the Vietnam War. In Perdita's case, it is a matter of her inability to testify on behalf of the Aboriginal people. Thus Roth and Jones deploy the stutter not only in gendered terms, as a symbol for the suppression of the female voice, but also like Graves, they deploy the condition as a broader symbol for the struggle to achieve political voice in the face of injustice.

In *American Pastoral*, Meredith "Merry" Levov is introduced as the "Rimrock Bomber," who in 1968 blows up the post office in Old Rimrock, inadvertently killing a town doctor and demolishing the adjacent general store.[36] As an intelligent child, Merry displays a stubborn streak and grows into an overweight, rebellious teenager, the "ugliest daughter ever born of two attractive parents."[37] Merry's father Seymour "Swede" Levov, a mythical athlete during his high school years in Newark, and her mother Dawn Dwyer, a former Miss New Jersey, are regarded as model parents by the small community of Rimrock and make every effort to provide their daughter with the proper treatment for her condition. Merry sees a speech therapist twice a week, keeps a diary in which she records the daily fluctuations of her stutter, and visits the local psychiatrist every Saturday.

At the age of 2, Merry tells her father that she feels "lonesome," a memory which later leads the Swede to suspect that what lies behind her speech troubles are "all those words she uncannily knew before other kids could pronounce their own names, the emotional overload of a vocabulary that included even 'I'm lonesome.'"[38] Merry's precociousness certainly heightens her awareness that her speech disorder separates her from other children her own age, but the suggested etiology of her stutter in the novel follows the predominant psychoanalytic view among speech pathologists of the 1940s and '50s that stuttering forms part of an unresolved Oedipal complex. In a meeting with the Swede, Merry's psychiatrist diagnoses her speech disorder as stemming specifically from her rivalry with her mother:

> It seemed that the etiology of Merry's problem had largely to do with her having such good-looking and successful parents. . . . [H]er parental good fortune was just too much for Merry, and so, to withdraw from the competition with her mother, to get her mother to hover over and focus on her and eventually climb the walls—and, in addition, to win the father away from the beautiful mother—she chose to stigmatize herself with a severe stutter, thereby manipulating everyone from a point of seeming weakness.[39]

This etiology closely parallels the kind of Oedipal reading offered by the influential Freudian speech pathologist Isador Coriat, who argued in the 1940s that female stutterers suffer from a castration complex in which, "the tongue has become a displaced phallus; the inner conflict with the libidinal economy has become concentrated on the lingual organ for the purpose of unconsciously satisfying a masculine aim . . . . Chronologically, the original castrator is the mother, and as a consequence female stammerers, as part of the Oedipus situation, hate their mothers."[40] With Merry, the psychiatrist believes that her stuttering signifies "an extremely manipulative, an extremely useful, if not even a vindictive type of behavior" meant to torment her mother.[41] In addition to the competition between mother and daughter, Merry frequently feels stifled by what her psychiatrist describes as her "highly pressured perfectionist family."[42] Unattractive and overweight, Merry can sense that she "doesn't quite measure up to Mother."[43] Though Merry is herself a perfectionist, her tireless efforts to correct her flawed speech prove futile, leaving her painfully aware that her "stuttering just killed her mother, and that killed Merry. 'I'm not the problem—Mother is!'"[44]

This idea of perfectionism is the theme around which Roth structures the three-part narrative of the Swede's Adamic fall from his idyllic life. Evoking both Genesis and Milton's epic, Roth titles the novel's three sections, "Paradise Remembered," "The Fall," and "Paradise Lost," through which the Swede stands as a Jewish-American Adam who creates "his version of paradise" in the form of the American pastoral.[45] Thanks to his flawless good looks and athletic prowess, the Newark Jewish community sees the Swede as the embodiment of their own hopes for assimilation. When the quasimythic Swede later marries a Catholic beauty queen, the novel's narrator Nathan Zuckerman marvels at how the Swede has indeed succeeded in achieving the assimilationist vision of the American dream. But when the Swede's beloved Merry destroys his seemingly innocent world by setting off the bomb that kills the local doctor, the question that continues to haunt the Swede is how he, with all "his carefully calibrated goodness," could still have produced "the angriest kid in America."[46] In his desperate attempt to pinpoint the original sin that propelled him and his family out of their Edenic paradise, the Swede agonizes over whether it was his daughter's imperfection in speech or some accidental flaw in his own parenting that turned her from a harmless stutterer into a terrorist bomber.

The incident that the Swede looks back on as his most serious "parental misstep" occurs when 11-year-old Merry, pretending to be a grown-up, playfully asks, "Daddy, kiss me the way you k-k-kiss umumumother."[47] By seeking an adult sexual relationship with her father, Merry is obviously enacting the Oedipal rivalry with the mother for the affection of the father. In response, the Swede uncharacteristically loses "his vaunted sense of proportion . . . and kisse[s] her stammering mouth with the passion that she had been asking for."[48] Though the kiss lasts only a few seconds, the Swede later questions whether this momentary lapse is what pushes Merry toward the aggressive behavior that culminates in her bombing the Rimrock post office. Almost overnight after their kiss, Merry becomes a "large, loping, slovenly sixteen-year-old," increasingly defiant and "angry because she stutters."[49] Deciding that "what was deforming her life wasn't the stuttering but the futile effort to overturn it," she not only ceases to follow normative speech patterns, but also rejects her privileged upbringing and seemingly perfect family life:

> The ridiculous significance she had given to that stutter to meet the Rimrock expectations of the very parents and teachers and friends who had caused her to so overestimate something as secondary as the way she talked. Not what she said but how she said it was all that bothered them. And all she really had to do to be free of it was to not give a shit about how it made them so miserable when she had to pronounce the letter *b*. . . . Vehemently she renounced the appearance and the allegiances of the good little girl

who had tried so hard to be adorable and loveable like all the other good little Rimrock girls—renounced her meaningless manners, her petty social concerns, her family's "bourgeois" values.[50]

The expectations placed on Merry to be a good little girl reflect the kind of social restraints on young girls of her era to be demure, both in conduct and in speech. Unlike with stuttering in men, where fluency is equated with masculine self-assertiveness, Roth suggests here that female stutterers are encouraged to attain fluency less for their own self-expression than for the purpose of maintaining a good appearance. Merry's father is of course a strict conformist, and his desire to maintain a perfect life leads his brother Jerry to accuse him of doing everything for the sake of appearances, even to the point of loving his daughter and wife as mere tokens of his assimilation into the American dream. Against her father's strong sense of decorum, Merry begins to use her stutter *performatively* as a means to resist and eventually attack her father's adherence to social norms. According to another Freudian speech pathologist I. Peter Glauber, the stutter has a secondary value in that it "can be used more or less consciously as a spiteful aggression against a parent who overvalues the function of speech."[51] Likewise, Merry's psychiatrist diagnoses her stutter as a vindictive response to her perfectionist parents who "tend to place an unrealistically high value on her every utterance."[52] Her decision to flaunt her stutter openly, to replace the effort of perfecting the sound of her words with the more meaningful endeavor of cultivating their substance, thus acts as a refusal to conform to her family's perfectionist demands.

Merry finds the ideal outlet for this newfound "freedom of speech" by channeling her stutter into overtly political forms of protest against what she views as the complicity of her father's generation in the Vietnam War:

> She had wasted enough time on the cause of herself. "I'm not going to spend my whole life wrestling day and night with a fucking stutter when kids are b-b-b-being b-b-b-b-bu-bu-bu roasted alive by Lyndon B-b-b-baines b-b-b-bu-bu-burn-'em-up Johnson!"
>
> All her energy came right to the surface now, unimpeded, the force of resistance that had previously been employed otherwise; and by no longer bothering with the ancient obstruction, she experienced not only her full freedom for the first time in her life but the exhilarating power of

total self-certainty. A brand-new Merry had begun, one who'd found, in opposing the "v-v-v-vile" war, a difficulty to fight that was worthy, at last, of her truly stupendous strength.[53]

It is interesting to note Roth's pun here on Merry's "unimpeded" energy in relation to the sudden release of her speech impediment. Rather than having Merry's newly liberated energy result in a spontaneous moment of fluency, Roth instead offers us the paradox of Merry *stuttering unimpeded*, that is to say, the obstruction which before prevented her from speaking freely now provides her with the very means of achieving full freedom to express herself. Merry becomes "f-f-f-free," in other words, not by being completely cured of her stutter, but on the contrary, by heightening its severity for rhetorical effect.[54] Roth emphasizes the intensity of Merry's need to express herself verbally, regardless of the acuteness of her stuttering in any given situation, by repeating the initial consonant of the stuttered word in an even more exaggerated fashion than one finds in standard depictions of stuttered speech, such as when Merry asks her father, "What *do* you b-b-b-b-b-b-b-believe in?"[55] When the Swede tries to stop her from participating in protest rallies, Merry's speech explodes into another angry outpouring of unimpeded energy: "This isn't a b-b-b-b-b-b-b-business . . . . What are you going to do? B-barricade me in? How are you going to stop me?"[56] In this way, Roth can be said to invert the stutter into something other than its conventional status as a sign of weakness or timidity. For Merry, it becomes an indicator of her newfound freedom, her "stupendous strength," and her weapon for resisting both gender and generational expectations.

Immersing herself in the antiwar movement, Merry quickly exhibits the first signs of the destructive behavior that will culminate in the bombing of the Rimrock post office. In her interactions with her family, she finds every opportunity to "*blast away* at the dinner table about the immorality of their bourgeois life" (emphasis added).[57] The more involved she becomes in antiwar protests, the more her family lives "in dread of [her] stuttering tongue."[58] Used as a weapon, her speech impediment is described as, "the machete with which to mow all bastard liars down. 'You f-f-fucking madman! You heartless mi-mi-mi-miserable m-monster!' she snarled at Lyndon Johnson whenever his face appeared on the seven o'clock news."[59] Again, whereas portrayals of male stutterers ordinarily emphasize weakness or nervousness as the defining character trait, the characteristic which defines Merry specifically as a stutterer is something the narrator Zuckerman terms the "stutterer's hatred of injustice," in other words, her stubbornly uncompromising morality.[60] This view of the stutterer corresponds closely to the analysis of the stuttering personality type put forward in 1937 by Robert West, the leading American speech pathologist of the first half of the twentieth century. In the foundational text of the field of American speech pathology, *The Rehabilitation of Speech*, West claims that the stutterer's most prominent personality trait is his moral rigidity:

> He is a perfectionist, not only in speech, but in all his conduct. He has an uncompromising conscience . . . . He makes moral issues out of every activity of his life . . . . He attaches moral significance even to his failures in speech, sometimes even regarding stuttering as a natural punishment for moral failure. In spite of his impediment in speech, he *must* express himself orally. Every failure in speech seems to increase his obligation to talk.[61]

As noted above, Merry is herself a perfectionist, especially in her initial efforts to correct her stutter. She works diligently, even as a child, on her stuttering diary, detailing her speech disorder in "page after page in her strikingly neat handwriting."[62] When she develops an intense passion for Audrey Hepburn, she spends the next several months imitating the actress's "light, crisp enunciation" in the hopes of curing herself.[63] Ultimately, Merry's perfectionist streak is replaced with a more dangerous form of moral rigidity, that is, her fanatical involvement in acts of terrorism.

Critics have tended to read Roth's portrayal of Merry's antiwar fanaticism as part of a change in attitude about 1960s radicalism to be found across his later works. Edward Alexander, for one, considers Merry as Roth's most condemnatory statement on 1960s leftists who abhor their parents' brand of liberalism, zealously spout radical political doctrines, and display a propensity toward violence.[64] Other critics, such as Sandra Stanley in her recent article on *American Pastoral*, have noted the sense of shared responsibility across the generations represented by Merry and the Swede for the rupture in what Stanley calls the "the mythic basis of the American dream."[65] Stanley goes on to suggest that while Roth is critical of Merry for being indiscriminately against everything, he is equally careful to remind us that the Swede's blind conviction in American myths contributes to Merry's uncontrollable rage.[66] What critics have almost universally glossed over, however, in readings of Merry's radicalism, is the symbolic weight of her stutter as the link between her early acts of political protests and her explosive violence. This underlying connection between political voice, stutter, and violence is made explicit within the novel by the Swede's brother Jerry, who tells him, "you made the angriest kid in America. Ever since she was a kid, every word she *spoke* was a bomb."[67] Jerry goes so far as to suggest that Merry's bombing is an act of retaliation against the world for her speech condition: "so to pay everybody back for her stuttering, she set off the bomb."[68] Moreover, the pejorative association between stuttered speech and violence is reinforced by the fact that Merry, as we are told, "never stuttered when she was with the dynamite."[69] Merry's paradoxically impeded/unimpeded speech thus allows her to achieve freedom by resisting her father's expectations. As such, the fluctuations between fluency and blocked speech in Merry stand as a measure of her relative success in resisting the silencing of her voice, an indication not of weakness or timidity but of stubborn strength. At the same time, the incoherence of her political ramblings can be said to offer a more conventional indictment of the chaotic nature of '60s radicalism, or what Roth calls "the counterpastoral . . . the indigenous American berserk."[70]

"haltings and erasures"

As her name suggests, the character of Perdita Keene in Gail Jones' recent novel *Sorry* represents another lost daughter from an equally tumultuous period in Australian history, the era of the Stolen Generations. Set in Western Australia during the early 1940s, the novel shifts between first and third person as Perdita recalls her lonely childhood raised by self-absorbed parents, English expatriates whose unsuccessful marriage is epitomized by the mutual neglect of their daughter. Perdita grows up in a household where "so much was hidden or unsaid," with a remote father who believes children should be seen and not heard and an unstable mother who takes refuge in the works of Shakespeare to escape her domestic responsibilities.[71] As such, Perdita is forced to become a "smallish adult," anxious for her parents' approval, but also "wilfully emphatic in ways [she] knew would test and annoy them," displaying both a stubbornness and a precociousness similar to those of Merry Levov.[72] Initially, Perdita's only source of affection comes from her Aboriginal wet nurse, but she later develops a close friendship with her neighbor's son Billy Trevor, a deaf mute who only speaks "through the wayward movements of his body," and with Mary, an Aboriginal girl taken from a convent to care for Perdita during Stella's bouts of depression at the hospital.[73] Jones' narrative is largely structured around the different responses to voicelessness that tie these three children together.

The etiology of Perdita's stutter differs from Merry's in that, as a young child, Perdita exhibits complete fluency in speech and describes herself as even once being a "flexible and canny speaker."[74] At the age of 10, however, she experiences "something that made her words seize and stick."[75] As Perdita explains the rarity of her own condition:

> Of all the anguishing forms of stutter that torment children (mostly males, as it happens, statistically, at least), mine was one of the rarer. Called psychogenic, it is the consequence of shock, or upset or circumstantial disaster. It is infrequent in its appearance and enigmatic in its cure. Most stuttering is developmental, and fades over time; the eruption of stuttering, as it were, is a stranger thing.[76]

Unlike Merry's stutter, which develops gradually and can only be alleviated through destruction, the sudden eruption of Perdita's speech disorder stems directly from the trauma of killing her father.

Returning from a visit with Billy, Perdita witnesses her father raping her Aboriginal caretaker Mary, and she reacts by stabbing him with a carving knife. To protect Perdita, Mary confesses to the crime, but the traumatic event causes Perdita to perform a "distinctive forgetting" in which she erases from her memory her own responsibility for her father's death and Mary's imprisonment.[77] The following morning, Perdita discovers at breakfast that "some trace of the violence remained like congestion in her mouth. . . . Something mangled her speech, syllables jammed."[78] The link established between Perdita's memory loss and her loss of fluency, what she collectively terms her "haltings and erasures," is rendered by Jones through a series of spatial images that together suggest Perdita lacks the necessary "room" to speak openly about what happened.[79] When signs of the stutter first appear, Perdita explains that her mother is convinced her speech disorder "was an affectation that I had developed to annoy her, or to dramatise my father's death in the very *chamber* of my mouth" (emphasis added).[80] The link between memory and language is epitomized in another spatial image of the house, the emblematic shape in which Perdita hides her secret:

> It is an image of our house, seen at night from outside, that I continually revisit . . . . Mr. Trevor had gone earlier to light the kerosene lamps, and as we came upon it, beneath a three-quarter moon, I saw emblematically the shape I would seal my secret within. I was already choked by words and inexpressive, I already had a cramped and mangled speech; here was the shape to contain my calamity.[81]

Jones' conception of space in this passage operates on two interrelated levels. First, Perdita's speech disorder is rendered in spatialized terms as the experience of a tongue that is too cramped to function properly. Second, it is the physical act of re-entering this traumatic space, of walking into the very room where the murder took place, that produces in Perdita the erasure of both memory and speech. Consequently, her speechlessness manifests throughout the novel as a kind of *shapelessness* in which any attempt to locate the true substance of the event creates a "dissolving of memory . . . a gap and shapelessness to her own lost history."[82] Perdita's troubled negotiation of suppressed memories and blocked speech is therefore ultimately a struggle to find the right space in which to give voice and shape to her words.

Not surprisingly, Perdita's memory loss leads her to decide that "silent words, not utterance, would be my form of expression."[83] Just as the etiologies of Merry's and Perdita's stutters are reversed, so too then is the manner in which they adapt to their condition. In contrast to Merry's project of revalorizing her stutter into an explosive form of protest against social constraints, Perdita internalizes her stutter, withdrawing into silence to such an extreme that she nearly loses her voice entirely. Before the onset of her speech disorder, Perdita is already well accustomed to silence due to the lack of communication between her parents, along with her father's expectation that she be seen and not heard (reminiscent of the pressure placed on Merry to conduct herself like a good little girl). With the onset of her condition, however, Perdita recognizes that her "ruined speech" reduces her to "a kind of object," to someone who is assumed to have nothing to say.[84] Her only source of escape comes through the "silent words of books" which offers her, again in spatialized terms, "a release, a flight" from the cramped chamber of stuttering.[85]

After the bombing of Dutch refugees by Japanese planes on 3 March 1942, Stella and Perdita are forced to flee Broome and move to Perth. By this stage in the novel, Perdita is virtually mute, and when her mother is again hospitalized for depression, Perdita goes to live with foster parents, Ted and Flora Ramsays, who provide her with the first real opportunity to find a cure for her speech disorder. To encourage Perdita to express herself more freely, Flora gives her a notebook in which she can write down her thoughts, and she embraces the "freedom to make her silence into another kind of text."[86]

Ironically, it is through the recitation of Shakespearean verse, her mother's chosen mode of escape, that Perdita finally achieves her first partial release from the confines of stuttering. For the first time, she finds in the language of Shakespeare, "a bright, fluent space I could play my voice in."[87] At the end of the school term, Perdita chooses to recite Hamlet's "To be or not to be" soliloquy, and her ability to speak unbroken Shakespeare is yet again likened to an openness of space accompanied by flight, as she hears her "voice swing upwards, unfastened, like a flying kite. For a while she was buoyed; she was in a dream of fluency. From her open mouth: flight."[88]

The treatment of her speech disorder is conducted by Doctor Victor Oblov, a Russian émigré and speech therapist who facilitates her eventual recovery of both speech and memory. Perdita conceives of Doctor Oblov's office as the metaphorical space she needs to recover: "Now there was this room in which a man . . . was unembarrassed and confiding, was sincerely interested in her story, a room in which–she believed it then–she would gradually relearn to speak."[89] The first form of speech therapy prescribed by Doctor Oblov is the recitation of iambic pentameter, through which she gradually learns to control her stutter by speaking in a "sing-song and exaggerated Shakespearean manner."[90] During the breakthrough scene with Doctor Oblov, Perdita is in the midst of reciting a scene from *Macbeth*, in order to "[loosen] the tongue," when she suddenly sees before her the exact series of events surrounding her father's death.[91] She remembers Mary's gaze before she stabs her father, she remembers Billy coming forward to remove the knife from her father's back, and finally, she remembers hearing Stella reciting the very same passage from *Macbeth*. This epiphantic moment of remembering coincides, as might be expected, with a complete recovery of her speech, as Perdita then proceeds to relate to Doctor Oblov in "unstuttering words" what she has just remembered: "It was like a biblical miracle to have a voice returned . . . . Perdita heard, to her amazement, her own verbal recovery. The knotted stutter was almost entirely gone, and instead words poured from her mouth, clear and even as water. Something had opened, released."[92]

The silencing of Perdita's voice is only one example of several suppressed voices struggling to find expression in *Sorry*. To politicize the condition of silence itself, Jones compiles a litany of marginal states of language to demonstrate the many ways in which individuals can be deprived of voice and forced to adapt through other means, in order to achieve some level of self-expression. Mary, for instance, has cultivated a multiplicity of voices through her skilled use of mimicry: "She shifted accents and registers; her tales held echoes and ironies. Perdita had never heard anyone speak so openly before, or, for that matter, in so many different voices."[93] Then, there is Billy's mutism and his adapting to his silence through the medium of sign language. Rejecting "the clumsy instrument of human speech," Billy teaches Perdita how to express herself instead through the "silent articulations of the body."[94] These variously marginal states of language, of voices being silenced and having to adapt into new forms of articulateness, gesture toward the specific historical events on which the title of Jones' novel is based. Between approximately 1910 and 1970, thousands of Aboriginal children were forcibly removed from their families and placed in government institutions or white foster homes. This historical injustice became the subject of a national inquiry in 1997, entitled *Bringing Them Home*, which compiled hundreds of eyewitness testimonies describing the large-scale removal of Aboriginal children, who are today known as the Stolen Generations. One year after the publication of this report, an annual National "Sorry Day" was declared, in spite of the Australian Government's refusal at that time to offer a formal apology.[95] To initiate a reconciliation process, the practice of signing "sorry books" was also launched to allow Australians to express their personal apologies to indigenous communities.

In her 2004 essay "Sorry-in-the-Sky," Jones elaborates how reflections on the Stolen Generations have only recently ushered Australia into what Shoshana Felman calls (in the context of trauma studies) the "age of testimony."[96] To articulate her own sense of the nature of testimony, Jones also turns to Cathy Caruth's notion of the unavoidable belatedness of any act of testifying. "Belatedness," writes Jones, "inheres in the incorrigible distance and dislocation of testimony."[97] Since the victim's unclaimed experience of trauma always exists in a distorted sense of temporality, the listener in turn experiences an unavoidable "delay and incompletion" in any reception of testimony.[98] This understanding of testimony as the inevitable experience of "belated utterance," for both speaker and listener, helps to clarify the role of the stutter in *Sorry* as a trope not just for a *lack* of speech, but also more importantly, for *belated* speech.[99] Initially, Perdita's dual loss of memory and speech is what prevents her from recognizing her responsibility to testify for Mary. After her recovery of fluency, however, Perdita finds herself trapped in yet another kind of speechlessness when she visits Mary and feels the impossibility of any kind of reparation for Mary's act of self-sacrifice. Perdita will only recognize much later, when she receives a letter informing her that Mary has died of appendicitis, that the day of her visit was the moment, "at which, in humility, she should have said 'sorry.'"[100] Much like the stutter she eventually overcomes, Perdita's lingering silence before Mary suffers from a tragic belatedness.

As I noted at the outset of this chapter, the association of blocked speech with destructiveness is an almost universal feature of fictional narratives about stuttering. From Billy Budd's lethal lashing out at Claggart in Melville's *Billy Budd* to Mizoguchi's burning down of the Golden Temple in Yukio Mishima's novel *Temple of the Golden Pavilion*, one finds the same model again and again in modern fiction of the nervous stutterer who, unable to assert himself through language, resorts to impulsive acts of aggression in order to alleviate his feeling of blockage.[101] While the characters of Merry and Perdita certainly adhere to this pejorative stereotype of the violent stutterer, their stories are complicated by the central issue of their gender. Roth and Jones are careful to remind us that these young girls suffer not so much from internal "maladies" as from the imposition of social norms, expectations, and the various familial relationships that disempower them. In this way, Roth and Jones expand the personal struggles of Merry and Perdita with fluency into the much broader issue of women's political voicelessness.

It is against this backdrop that we can best understand how Roth and Jones negotiate gender, politics, and history in their novels. Participation in the *vox populi*, for girls like Merry and Perdita, requires first a renegotiation of their place within a set of private family relationships. Ultimately, neither girl finds adequate resolution to the disempowerment they experience within the family by articulating their points of view outside the family. Merry's stutter represents an entire generation's inability to effectively articulate its opposition to the war, a failure which for Roth results in ever-escalating forms of violence.[102] Similarly, Perdita's persistent silence before Mary represents another generation's failure to speak up on behalf of the Aborigines, public testimony thought to suffer inevitably from the same belatedness as stuttered speech.

Tourettic Speech in Jonathan Lethem's *Motherless Brooklyn*

"Hence the necessity of speech and song; hence these throbs and heart-
beatings in the orator, at the door of the assembly, to the end, namely, that
thought may be ejaculated as Logos or Word. Doubt not, O poet, but persist.
Say, 'It is in me, and shall out.' Stand there, balked and dumb, stuttering and
stammering, hissed and hooted, stand and strive, until at last rage draw out
of thee that dream power which every night shows thee in thine own."

– Ralph Waldo Emerson, "The Poet"

"la maladie des tics"

Ideas about the root cause of Tourette's syndrome have undergone a series of changes in the past two centuries, and that series exactly mirrors the historical trajectory sketched in this book: starting with spiritual ideas about the cause of language breakdown, then moving from volitional theories to neurological to psychopathological (which is then further refined to psychosexual) before finally returning to the neurological. Evidence of undiagnosed cases of Tourette's syndrome stretches back to the Middle Ages, with their link to the strange phenomena of Saint Vitus' Dance (or Sydenham's chorea), a chaotic and uncontrollable form of movement usually coupled with glossolalic outbursts, which was believed to be caused by spiritual possession. By the eighteenth century, the jerky and stereotypic movements of a figure like Samuel Johnson, along with his occasional copralalic mutterings, were taken by his friends not as signs of demonic or divine possession but simply as part of the writer's eccentricity and his potentially pending madness. Since then, of course, reports of Doctor Johnson's ticcishness have been posthumously diagnosed as a textbook case of Tourette's. Throughout the nineteenth century, the shifting views on another famous case highlight the dramatic changes in scientific understandings of motor and vocal tics, again, changes that adhere closely to the ways in which conditions like aphasia, mutism, and stuttering were understood. The case in question involved the sad and scandalous lifestory of the Marquise de Dampierre, first reported in 1825 by the French physician Jean Marc Gaspard Itard. In addition to her bodily tics, Itard noted the frequent and uncontrollable copralalic outbursts that made the Marquise a pariah in Parisian social circles and eventually forced her to retreat into total seclusion:

> All of a sudden, without being able to prevent it, she interrupts what she is saying or what she is listening to with bizarre shouts and with words that are even more extraordinary and which make a deplorable contrast with her intellect and her distinguished manners. These words are for the most part gross swear words and obscene epithets and, something that is no less embarrassing for her than for the listeners, an extremely crude expression of a judgment or of an unfavorable opinion of someone in the group.[1]

In his book *A Cursing Brain?: The Histories of Tourette Syndrome*, Howard Kushner demonstrates how Itard's report of this notorious case was revisited throughout the nineteenth century and essentially rediagnosed secondhand by numerous clinicians who had encountered patients presenting with similarly mysterious symptoms. The eponymous discoverer of the condition, Georges Gilles de la Tourette, would not reevaluate the case of the Marquise until 1885, as part of his landmark case study "Étude sur une affection nerveuse caracterisée par de l'incoordination motrice accompagneé d'echolalie et de coprolalie," published in the *Archives de Neurologie*.[2] Between Tourette's account and that of Itard, one finds several doctors who understood ticcishness in what we might call Melvillean terms, as a failure or disease of the will itself. In 1847, Ernest Billod argued as much in his *Maladies de la Volonté*, citing the case of the Marquise, whom he had never treated himself, as proof of his view that the will was a kind of physical organ which could be damaged by lesions. What the Marquise had suffered from, according to Billod, was "a *lesion* of association of ideas, of memory, of reminiscence, and of imagination," which prevented her from restraining her frequent fits of cursing.[3] Building on Billod's study, Theodule Ribot took up the Marquise's case in his own 1883 study, also titled *Les Maladies de la Volonté*, using her as an example of what he called "the idiocy of the will" when the impairment is severe enough to remove the patient's ability of self-restraint.[4]

Two years later, Charcot would encourage his pupil George Gilles de la Tourette to publish a report on the various cases of this malady of tics Tourette had been compiling from all over the globe, among which was included the posthumous case study of the Marquise de Dampierre. For Tourette, the most difficult hurdle came in convincing his peers that these seemingly unrelated symptoms had a single root cause. Convinced they did, Tourette hypothesized that the etiology of these various symptoms was firmly neurological, and his arguments for the organic basic of the syndrome which now bears his name placed him in a position similar to that of Paul Broca with respect to the reception Broca's theory of cerebral localization initially received in the early 1860s. The response to Tourette's "Étude," especially by many of Charcot's other students, was perhaps even more harsh than the backlash against Broca's view of the cerebral basis of language and language loss. Most of the skepticism was directed at the classification itself, over whether Tourette had truly uncovered a discrete illness or had simply cobbled together various unrelated symptoms under a single heading. There were other critics who did agree with Charcot that Tourette had in fact discovered a new illness but disagreed over the proposed cause. As Kushner notes, "many of Charcot's colleagues and students were convinced that Gilles de la Tourette's classification was, instead, a florid manifestation of hysteria."[5] In these initial criticisms of Tourette's etiology, we can see how the syndrome begins to follow an identical path to that of stuttering: from neurological to psychoneurotic to psychosexual.

It is often pointed out that Tourette's syndrome then fell off the medical map for several decades after its controversial first appearance in 1885, not resurfacing until 1969 when the famous dopamine experiments of doctors like Oliver Sacks brought the condition back into prominence. Most research that was done on tics in the decades after 1885, by clinicians like Edouard Brissaud (whose influence on Proust has already been noted), Meige, and

Feindel, portrayed the Ticcer in what will by this point be highly familiar psychopathological terms, as someone whose speech was disturbed by their neurotic personality type.[6] The only difference from the Stutterer, in this regard, was that their neurosis was said to produce a *failure* of inhibition, a hyperactivity which often took socially inappropriate forms, as opposed to the hyperinhibition associated with stuttering. Shortly after World War I, just as with theories of stuttering, psychogenic accounts of the Ticcer, according to Kushner, "segued into Freudian explanations of early childhood sexual repressive conflict."[7] The leading proponent of the psychosexual view will come as no surprise either. In 1921, Sandor Ferenczi claimed that tics were an unconscious reenactment of repressed masturbatory urges.[8] Just as the Stutterer's intermittent speech was an outward manifestation of his inner longing for the maternal nipple, so too the Ticcer's jerky movements were nothing other than a sublimated expression of autoerotic impulses, or as Ferenczi put it, "the stereotyped equivalents of Onanism."[9]

Tourette's would then virtually disappear from medical and social discourses until the 1970s, and it only began to attain a level of social visibility equal to the other speech disorders studied in this work after the famous experimental treatments conducted by doctors like Oliver Sacks at Mount Carmel Hospital in 1969. In his 1973 book *Awakenings*, Sacks describes his attempt to treat catatonic patients through the administering of synthetic dopamine (L-Dopa), and the tourettic or Parkinson-like effects of hyperactivity, saccadic movements, and palilalia that it produced in his patients. The discovery that the neurotransmitter dopamine played a central role in conditions that would seem to be polar opposites of one another, catatonia and ticcishness, made it undeniable that Tourette was right to posit an organic basis for his syndrome, and it is now understood almost universally as a neurological disorder located in the basal ganglia region of the brain.

With respect to the literary representation of Tourette's syndrome which will be the topic of this chapter, the distinction Oliver Sacks makes in *The Man Who Mistook His Wife for a Hat* between pathologies of deficit and pathologies of excess is especially helpful here. Deficit, Sacks points out, is "neurology's favorite word" because of the field's fundamentally mechanistic view of our vocal and physical capacities.[10] In the case of language, there is either deficit or there is function. Either dysfluency or fluency. But in his writings on Tourette's, Sacks also explores deficit's opposite: "What then of its opposite—an excess of or superabundance of function? Neurology has no word for this—because it has no concept. A function, or functional system, works—or it does not: these are the only possibilities it allows. Thus a disease which is 'ebullient' or 'productive' in character challenges the basic concepts of neurology."[11] Tourette's syndrome is one such disease for Sacks, a condition which, when treated and rechanneled properly, can lead to staggering amounts of creativity and artistic output.

The distinction between deficit and excess is particularly relevant to an understanding of the type of language breakdown represented by tourettic speech. The involuntary verbal tics and copralalic outbursts common to sufferers of Tourette's syndrome offer an altogether different version of breakdown from those treated in Chapters 1–4. From a clinical standpoint, of course, the distinction must be maintained between aphasic disorders that disrupt the language faculty itself and speech-fluency disorders such as stuttering and lisping which affect only the proper articulation of words. However, in their fictional portrayal, as we have found, the differences among these conditions (both in cause and symptom) become less important than their underlying meaning as sociocultural symbols. What they have in common is an understanding of the breakdown of language as something that stems from the speaker's inability to *actively* or *freely* produce words. We have already seen the issues of willpower and temperament that arise from this, not only in the cases of stutterers like Billy Budd and Billy Bibbit, whose weakness as men is used to account for their intermittent speech, but even in the case of the mutism of a Madame Raquin, where it is ultimately her will-to-speak (and not her brain) that is said to fail her. By contrast, the phonic tics of tourettic speech represent an entirely opposite form of dysfluency. Tourettic speech is not an inability to produce words, but an inability to *restrain* the production of words. Rather than the absence of language, what we will find instead in this final disorder is an absence of restraint, and the resulting flow of language in a state of uncontrollable excess.

"the world (or my brain – same thing)"

The narrator of Jonathan Lethem's *Motherless Brooklyn*, Lionel Essrog, repeatedly uses metaphors of fluidity to describe the excessive quality of his own verbal production. Language, for Lionel, is always "spilling out of me unrestrained."[12] The source of his tourettic utterances is "a sea of language . . . reaching full boil" inside him.[13] This fluid excess, however, is not seen by Lionel through Sacks' rose-colored glasses, as a creative overflow, but rather as a destabilizing force, too powerful to hold back, that fights its way out of him: "So I kept my tongue wound in my teeth, ignored the pulsing in my cheek, the throbbing in my gullet, persistently swallowed language back like vomit."[14] The progression of Tourette's syndrome in Lionel's case can be said to follow a fairly typical pattern, with the onset of motor tics preceding verbal ones by a period of several years.[15] Lionel's earliest memory of ticcing involves a visit to the Natural History Museum in Manhattan during which he sneaks into one of the dioramas to caress a penguin and then proceeds to touch each and every penguin inside the display in a compulsive form of the children's game of tag. "Once I'd touched the first penguin," he concedes, "I had no choice."[16] The frequency of his tics quickly increases following the penguin incident so that a mere 9 months later, now age 12, Lionel notes, "I had begun to overflow with reaching, tapping, grabbing, and kissing urges— those compulsions emerged first, while language for me was still trapped like a roiling ocean under a calm floe of ice."[17] By the age of 13, his tourettic energy has found "other outlets, other obsessions," and he develops what he describes as a proneness, in his particular case, "to floor-tapping, whistling, tongue-clicking, winking, rapid head turns, and wall-stroking, anything but the direct utterances for which my particular Tourette's brain most yearned. Language bubbled inside me now, the frozen sea melting, but it felt too dangerous to let out."[18] At this early stage, Lionel would seem to have already developed his first coping skill, the rechanneling of his tourettic energy into more socially acceptable forms, that is, until his urge to maintain a constant contact with the outside world takes the form of kissing and groping other boys in his orphanage where he grows up.

By the starting point of the narrative, when Lionel along with his disease has reached full maturity, he still presents with this constant urge to reestablish contact with his environment through a variety of physical tics. He also exhibits a perhaps slightly higher than normal evidence of related obsessive compulsive behaviors, along with a relatively low incidence of copralalia. Overall, his symptomatology could be described as a fairly normal case, however, Lionel is quick to remind us that one of the defining features of Tourette's is its especially strong resistance to generalizations. Even more so than with other syndromes, the combination of tourettic behaviors is always unique to each tourettic self because, while the urge to respond to one's environment may be compelled, the form of that response is usually not. Lionel first becomes aware of the fact that his disease will always be experienced as *my* disease (and his brain as "my particular Tourette's brain") when his benefactor Frank Minna buys him a book called *Understanding Tourette's Syndrome.*[19] Reading the book, Lionel sardonically reports, enabled him to contextualize his symptoms and in the process to appreciate how, "my constellation of behaviors was 'unique as a snowflake,' oh, joy, and evolving, like some microscoped crystal in slow motion, to reveal new facets."[20] This same point is made by Oliver Sacks in his account of a surgeon's ticcishness from *An Anthropologist on Mars.* According to Sacks, one of the things that makes ticcing so fascinating, not just medically but culturally, is its liminal status between voluntary and involuntary action, or between meaningful and meaningless behaviors:

Tics can have an ambiguous status, partway between meaningless jerks or noises and meaningful acts. Though the tendency to tic is innate in Tourette's, the particular *form* of tics often has a personal or historical origin. Thus a name, a sound, a visual image, a gesture, perhaps seen years before and forgotten, may first be unconsciously echoed or imitated and then preserved in the stereotypic form of a tic.[21]

For Lionel, this insight that his tics are a personalized response to his environment provides little more than cold comfort, a feeble message of empowerment for someone who feels imprisoned in his symptoms. The therapeutic intention of this type of message may be to alleviate the patient's feelings of isolation and stigmatization by instead focusing on how the uniqueness of his condition individualizes him. But Lionel feels that his tics, rather than making him "unique as a snowflake," only individualize the disease itself. In other words, his symptoms merely bestow a distinct personality on his tourettic brain.[22]

To emphasize this throughout the novel, Lethem employs the device of personification to portray his brain virtually as another character with the ability to act, think, and speak independently from within Lionel. What we might call this novel's neural fallacy—Lionel's attributing of a distinct agency to his tourettic Self set apart from his other Self—is articulated in terms of a "double brain," or "my two disgruntled brains," forced like an odd couple to cohabitate in the same space.[23] Lionel constantly feels himself divided between his tourettic and his nontourettic selves, with each part functioning simultaneously on different tracks. When he contemplates the scant clues behind his mentor Frank Minna's death, for instance, he observes that, "while I thought about these things, another track in my brain intoned brainyoctomy brainyalimony bunnymonopoly baileyoctopus brainyanimal broccopotamus."[24] As such, his experience of his own mind (though "mind" is the wrong word in this context) is always a matter of division and compartmentalization, of negotiation between two disgruntled parties, his normal self and his unruly brain.[25] One can imagine what a more conventional rendering of this experience of multilayered consciousness would look like, expressed in terms of semiconscious thoughts in the "back" of one's mind. In this formulation, the same mental compartmentalization would occur, but the separate tracks or spaces of consciousness would still allow for the supervenience of a governing, unified, thinking self. But in Lionel's case, the supervenience of the diseased brain over the self is underscored by the grammatical positioning of "my brain" as the active subject performing its action (i.e. intoning, thinking, puzzling, keeping watch, saying, etc.). Lethem's stock phrase for signaling that the tourettic self has taken over is the personified formulation: "My brain went . . . ." By virtue of this neural construction, Lionel stands more as a witness to what his brain is doing independently of himself than as some Cartesian *res cogitans* who thinks *with* his brain. This fragmented experience of consciousness almost reaches the point of a split personality disorder, in that he is regularly engaged in a kind of dialogue with his speaking brain, pleading at points for his tourettic self not to tic, and addressed in turn by this other pathological self inside him.[26]

The fact that Lionel's condition is understood in explicitly neurological terms, as a disease of the brain, situates *Motherless Brooklyn* in the same Naturalist tradition of Zola's *Thérèse Raquin*, and Lethem's novel can be seen as a revival of the neurophysiologically informed project articulated by Zola in both his 1867 Preface to *Thérèse Raquin* and his 1880 essay "Le Roman expérimental." As discussed in Chapter 1, Zola's goal was to compose a novel in which the material brain (as opposed to some higher faculty like the mind) is used to account for the characters' thoughts and actions. Zola's desire to replace traditional spiritual or psychological categories (mind, soul, conscience) with purely physiological ones (brain, nerves, blood) is apparent in his own consistent use of a neurophysiological vocabulary to explain human behavior throughout *Thérèse Raquin*.[27] Although Zola and Lethem both present their characters' higher faculties (soul, mind, language) in reductionist terms as neurological phenomena, Lionel's brain is also staged in a completely opposite way from that of Thérèse and Laurent. By the end of Zola's novel, Thérèse and Laurent have become unified as biological organisms who share a single brain, resulting in a physical intersubjectivity due to the mixing of their nerves and blood together. Lionel's more postmodern subjectivity, on the other hand, manifests itself as always already fragmented, doubled, in conflict with itself. He is a single but un-unified self consisting of mutually independent parts that move in and out of his control.

The strange mixture of "Kaos and Control," of involuntary and voluntary activity, that characterizes Lionel's tourettic condition finds another precedent in Zola's portrayal of the struggle between free will and determinism that marks Laurent's attempts at artistic production.[28] After Camille's death, Laurent's sanguine temperament grows more and more enervated by its contact with Thérèse's nervous temperament, resulting in his brief transformation into an artistic genius. What makes Laurent's neurophysiological transformation so strange is that for an artistic genius, Laurent's talent is extremely limited. He is only capable of painting a single subject, Camille's face. In any other novel, this would be considered the manifestation of Laurent's unconscious guilt, but Zola insists that the motor activity of painting the same face again and again is physiologically based and therefore involuntary. It is, in other words, an artistic tic. In Chapter 25, the narrator describes Laurent's attempt to stop sketching the image of Camille's drowned head. He consciously sets out to paint other subjects—the faces of angels, women, Roman warriors, animals—but his hand "kept tracing out the features of that dreadful face."[29] In what becomes a desperate attempt to determine "whether or not he was in control of his own hand," Laurent "fought against the compulsion that was directing his fingers.[30] With each new attempt he came back to the drowned man's face. However strongly he exerted his will to avoid the lines he knew so well, they were the ones he kept drawing, as, despite himself, he obeyed the promptings of his rebellious nerves and muscles."[31] Despite Laurent's repeated attempts to exert a higher will, his own nerves and muscles compel him to retrace Camille's features on the canvas, suggesting that even artistic genius or inspiration is understood deterministically or, we might say, ticcishly, as the involuntary performance of a given form.[32] The equivalents to Laurent's physical compulsions in *Motherless Brooklyn* are Lionel's "fifteen years of taps and touches," his compulsion to reach for things around him from shoulders to shirt collars to glove compartments, which are similarly described in terms of the futility of willpower in the face of his disease.[33] Lionel is acutely aware that even his voluntary gestures can ticcify themselves, that is, immediately and unavoidably convert from voluntary action to involuntary echopraxia: "I shrugged, palms up, toward the roof of the Lincoln. The gesture ticcified instantly, and I repeated it, shrug, palms flapped open, grimace."[34] Just as Laurent witnesses his hand asserting its own will over him, so too Lionel views his personified brain as an autonomous being exerting its control over his actions.

The neurological and deterministic similarities between *Thérèse Raquin* and *Motherless Brooklyn* also extend to Zola's and Lethem's similar approaches to the effect of environment on the individual. In Zola's novel, after Laurent experiences the neurophysiological process of enervation in which his blood adopts his lover's nerves, he comes to represent a new social type of modern urban life, what Zola calls the "new individual." The "new individual," or "nervous being," is a category that functions at once socially and medically, in that Laurent's transformation from hedonistic peasant to neurotic artist is also triggered by the overstimulation, or "enervation," of his new urban setting. Likewise in *Motherless Brooklyn*, Lionel is conscious of how the urban environment of New York, what he refers to as the "Tourettic city," reifies his tourettic brain.[35] In a postmodern and pathologized version of nineteenth-century flânerie, Lionel lets his physical tics lead him through the streets in what he calls "navigation by Tourette's."[36] For the most part though, Lionel's movement through New York is limited to a repeated series of controlled responses to urban signs, such as the stop and go of street lights. The many moments of driving, tailing, and weaving through city traffic can therefore be read together as an extended metaphor for Lionel's own experience of relative control. Lionel's ambulation is overdetermined by the involuntary on/off effect of his physical and verbal tics. He reacts compulsively to his surroundings, and the experience of responding to the city's spasmodic signals is indistinguishable from the jerky repetitions of Lionel's echopraxic behavior. It becomes clear that Lionel himself is conscious of these affinities between his syndrome and the urban environment when he watches the timed stoplights and jokes, "Now there . . . was a job for someone with obsessive-compulsive symptoms—traffic management."[37] For the same reason, he uses the metaphor of traffic to explain the relative lack of control that comes with his condition. "There's a lot of traffic in my head," Lionel notes, "and it's two-way."[38] It is here that the exact sense of the novel's other reductively neural refrain—"the world (or my brain – same thing)"[39]—starts to make itself clear. Lionel's experience of his inner tourettic brain and his outer surroundings are identical matters of "traffic," experiences of relative agency where one is only free to move under certain restrictions, restrictions that are partly contingent (the presence of others) and partly predictable (timed streetlights).

"to tic freely"

Although *Motherless Brooklyn* and *Thérèse Raquin* both prioritize the brain over more traditional faculties like the psyche or the mind, the key difference between their two Naturalisms is that Lionel is the narrator of his story and provides his own diagnosis of the machinations of his tourettic brain. In *Thérèse*

Raquin, the characters' psychological thoughts (as well as their supernatural hallucinations) exist at odds with the narrator's interventions, which serve to remind us of the biological determinism underlying the characters' ultimately false experiences of themselves and their situations. Thérèse and Laurent may understand their emotions, behaviors, and experiences in quasispiritual or psychological terms, but what Zola posits as the neurophysiological causes of their condition remain entirely opaque to them. By contrast, Lionel is acutely conscious that what he calls his "Personalityness" is largely a byproduct of his neurophysiology, in a way and to an extent that uneducated characters in a nineteenth-century novel simply could not be.[40] Presuming a highly nuanced awareness of the complexities of cause and effect behind his Tourette's, Lionel makes extremely fine distinctions about his symptoms and gauges precisely how controlled he is at any given moment. He distinguishes, for example, between tic-free moments, semicompulsive acts when he "wasn't *exactly* ticcing" (emphasis added), and moments when he is "tic-gripped, helpless," and the compulsion is so strong that he has "no choice" whatsoever.[41] Even the most subtle states of his tourettic condition appear to be transparent to him. After his second visit to the Zendo, for instance, Lionel observes that he "wasn't ticcing *much*, for a *couple of reasons*" (emphasis added).[42] The distinctions that Lionel makes here suggest both a qualitative and quantitative awareness (not ticcing "much") as well as a knowledge of various possible causes for when and why he is ticcing ("for a couple of reasons"). The specific "reasons" for his reduced ticcishness in this particular scene are first, that Kimmery's presence acts as an "unprecedented balm" to his nervousness, and second, the chaos of his day with its "tumult of unsorted clues" that give the "extra track in [his] brain . . . plenty of work to do threading the beads together."[43]

Like most of the stutterers we have examined, Lionel's "tics were always worst when [he] was nervous," and though Lionel usually sees himself as a "prisoner of [his] syndrome," he is nonetheless mindful of the ways in which his tics can be modified, made improvisational, even if his efforts to remaster them often prove unsuccessful.[44] This strategy of modification takes the form of a paradoxical desire to *tic voluntarily*, reminiscent of Merry Levov's ability to *stutter unimpeded* in *American Pastoral*. When sitting at gunpoint late in the novel, he suddenly "wanted to tic just for the hell of it."[45] In line with

Sacks' understanding of ticcishness as a complex mixture of improvisation and imprisonment, Lionel, in a confrontation with Tony prior to Minna's death, compulsively repeats the word "Dickweed" until he manages by "refining a verbal tic to free [himself] from its grip."[46] Lionel's attempt here not to stop, but to fine-tune his tic suggests again that acute awareness he claims to possess of the minute adjustments he undergoes from powerlessness to relative control. These moments where his understanding of his condition expands beyond the neurological stand out as exceptions to the overall rule. When Lionel finds himself "tongue-tied for once" in Kimmery's presence during their argument over Gerard Minna's real identity, Lionel begins "ticcing out of sheer frustration."[47] Though Lionel is usually at the mercy of his tourettic brain, at this particular moment, he becomes aware that his condition is not limited exclusively to neurological causes, but that psychogenic frustrations can also trigger his tics. This begs the same question posed by critic Lilian Furst with regard to Zola, that is, exactly how compatible this kind of naturalism is with the Novel as a genre. In the case of *Thérèse Raquin*, no matter how zealous Zola was to eliminate psychologism in the novel, he does fall back on a traditional psychologism at times. Similarly, in *Motherless Brooklyn*, Lionel's ability to account for his own condition in a purely neurological and deterministic way still allows for exceptions, moments where free will would seem to override pathology. Like Merry, Lionel struggles to understand what it would mean "to tic freely," and to find ways of doing so.[48]

This mixture of free will and determinism is most aptly encapsulated in the catchword "Freefreak!," something which Lionel shouts in response to Frank's comment that he is a free (in the monetary sense) "human freak show."[49] As a "Freefreak," Lionel is simultaneously a "Freakboy," compelled to act on his impulses, and yet free enough to choose the form in which his compulsions will take.[50] The oxymoronic sense of controlled chaos in this is made further symbolic with Lionel's place of employment, the Minna Agency, another obvious pun on the diminished ("Minna") agency of his tourettic self. Furthermore, the clandestine nature of his work at the "Agency" often means that he is required to carry out orders without knowing the reasons behind them, for instance, when the Minna men are told to destroy the Ferris wheel at a traveling Hispanic carnival: "This was the Agency at its mature peak:

unquestioning and thorough in carrying out an action even when it bordered on sheer Dada."[51] For Lionel, the Agency's nonsensical orders to engage in pointless activities offer yet another mirror in which to view his own ticcish behaviors, which also serve no purpose other than to obey the random orders of his brain.

To demonstrate how all of this relates to the issue of disordered speech, I will now lay out the elaborate system of willed and unwilled language that Lethem creates in *Motherless Brooklyn*. In the period before Lionel's disease finally progresses into verbal ticcishness, language is experienced as a force to be stifled and contained. For as long as he can, Lionel rechannels his urge to verbal outbursts into physical tics: "I collected words, treasured them like a drooling sadistic captor, bending them, melting them down, filing off their edges, stacking them into teetering piles, before release I translated them into physical performance, manic choreography."[52] Gradually, he loses this contest, and when his disease assumes its full verbal form, his tourretic brain acquires its own voice independent of Lionel. Lethem's method for rendering this double-voicedness is to use italics to distinguish between the two major modes of discourse in the novel, voluntary and involuntary. These two modes are doubled again, through the use of quotation marks, into interior thoughts and externalized utterances. Throughout the novel, this results in a seemingly chaotic but ultimately stable orthographical code, where Lionel's involuntary verbal tics, whether spoken or thought, are clearly separated from his more intentional utterances.

The most common form his tourettic speech takes in the novel is the sudden and embarrassing interruption of a voluntary utterance made by his brain: "I like you too Julia. There's nothing—*Screwtony! Nertscrony! Screwtsony! Tooscrewny!*—sorry. There's nothing wrong with that."[53] Based on Lethem's orthographical markers, one is able to distinguish the exact moment when control over the spoken dialogue shifts from Lionel to his tourettic brain. The same process of interruption applies internally to Lionel's unexpressed thoughts. The involuntary appearance of ticced thoughts, in a sense spoken by a distinct tourettic voice inside his multilayered head, raises interesting questions about how interior thought and language are typically rendered in the Modernist versus Postmodernist Novel. There is a longstanding debate among novel theorists, taken up by Dorothy Hale in relation to the work of Faulkner among others, over what exactly the relationship should be between a character's internal form of expression and his or her external manner of speaking.[54] Some of these critics have argued that for any narration of interiority to achieve authenticity, a character's private thoughts should be tonally approximate to his external mode of discourse. In short, characters should think more or less like they talk. Others in this debate have argued that privacy is a constitutive feature of our interiority, and there is therefore no reason why a character's interior monologue should not differ from the way he or she speaks in public. Lethem's novel is situated in a unique position in relation to this debate in that Tourette's syndrome can be said to impossibilize any rigid distinctions between internal and external forms of expression. The nature of Tourette's syndrome is such that Lionel's interiority is constantly being forced outward. For that very reason, Lionel's verbal tics are regularly presented as a struggle to keep his internal tics from being externalized, and his speech is thus perforated by ticcish words that are said to be swallowed, kept in check, held inside, or choked back to prevent them from being blurted out.[55] Rigid distinctions between internal and external forms of expressions, that is, between private thought and public language, become especially problematic when one examines the complex nature of Lionel's internal tics. As I have already noted, Lionel's brain is said to work on multiple tracks simultaneously. This is nothing unique to the sufferer of Tourette's, of course, but his feelings of powerlessness mean that it is experienced not as a wandering mind but as a never-ending "interior babble" speaking at him and over which he has no control.[56] The end result is a feeling of profound alienation from his own consciousness. Although Lionel is at least able to detach himself by reporting on his brain's musings, he is ultimately powerless to silence this second tourettic voice inside him. The interior ramblings of *Motherless Brooklyn* are further relevant to the novelistic debate over the proper tonality of interior monologue inasmuch as they gradually resemble a pathologized version of standard modernist stream-of-consciousness. In those moments when this touretticized stream-of-consciousness externalizes itself as involuntary utterance, any possible distinction between Lionel's private and public self is thrown into question. Unable to dictate the terms on which his interiority is made public, Lionel's tourettic language "spreads from its place at my private core to cover my surface, my public front."[57]

Lethem's neural refrain for signaling the shift from conscious thought to interior babble—"My brain went . . ."—is followed in each case by a string of verbal tics that vary in tone and duration from short relatively coherent utterances to circuitously repetitive utterances (reminiscent of the poetry of Gertrude Stein), to improvisational riffing on the speech of others (closer to the performative wordplay of African American signifyin') to an anagrammatical kind of nonsense language (not unlike the neologistic wordplay of Joyce's *Finnegans Wake*). These forms of linguistic disturbance can be roughly classified into three major types: (1) an anagrammatical form of nonsense language that often resembles voluntary wordplay, (2) mimicry of the speech of others, and (3) copralalic utterances.

At the beginning of the novel, when Lionel waits in the car for Minna's return, his brain interjects a fairly intelligible ticcish rambling: "My brain went *Follow that car! Hollywood star! When you wish upon a cigar!*"[58] Later at the hospital, his brain interrupts his thoughts again, but this time the internal tic is much more convolutedly repetitive, in the style, if we can call his tourettic thoughts a style, of Gertrude Stein: "I gritted my teeth while my brain went, *Guy walks into the ambulance ramp stabs you in the goddamn emergency gut says I need an immediate stab in the garbage in the goddamn walk-in ambulance says just a minute looks in the back says I think I've got a stab in the goddamn walk-in immediate ambuloaf ambulamp octoloaf oafulope.*"[59] Occasionally, Lionel's brain will make more creative analogical leaps, such as when Kimmery offers Lionel some Thai chicken soup and his brain immediately begins to free-associate: "*Tie-chicken-to-what?* went my brain. *Tinker to Evers to Chicken,*" an allusion to the great double-play trio of the Chicago Cubs, Tinker, Evers, and Chance.[60] Finally, there are Lionel's many internal babblings that take place inside his brain and that will ring familiar to readers of Joyce's *Finnegans Wake*: "My brain went, *Tourette's slipdrip stinkjet's blessdroop mutual-of-overwhelm's wild kissdoom.*"[61] Even when Lionel manages to express himself to others in a firmly controlled, intentional speech, he is still aware of and distracted by the "background of [his] own interior babble" going on inside his brain.[62] He experiences this internal babbling, for example, when a homicide detective questions his and Julia's alibis for Frank's murder. On the one hand, Lionel attempts to answer the detective's questions without ticcing aloud, while on the other hand, his brain simultaneously performs its own internal tic: "*Alibi hullabaloo gullible bellyflop smellafish*, sang my brain, obliterating speech."[63] Lionel's involuntary speech is clearly marked here through the use of italics, and the absence of quotation marks indicates that the tic is not spoken aloud, but held within himself.

In addition to the internal babbling of his brain, Lionel's involuntary tics also fall under the second category of mimicry. His physical tics frequently manifest as imitations of other characters' facial expressions and bodily gestures, while his verbal tics will sometimes adopt the sound of another's voice. This reversal of the ventriloquizing we found in stuttering is most often applied to Frank Minna, whose death leads Lionel to appropriate Frank's voice: "*I'll die when I'm dead,* my brain recited in Minna's voice."[64] During his drive to Maine, Lionel also finds himself hearing "Minna's voice now in place of my incessant tourettic tongue, saying, *Floor it, Freakshow. You got something to do, do it already,*" almost as though his Tourette's has given him the power to channel voices of the dead.[65] In both of these examples, the absence of quotation marks in the original text indicates that these italicized words are internally ticced by Lionel's tourettic brain, which is not only able to assert its own voice but also to mimic the voices of others.

Lionel's anagrammatism often involves a combination of the first two of the three modes we have delineated, where the reordering of letters is performed on words initially spoken by someone else. For instance, when Julia exclaims in disgust that she is the "heir to a corrupt and inept detective agency," Lionel's brain ticcishly riffs to itself, "*Inupt and corrept.*"[66] In a more linguistically ambiguous moment in the novel, when Lionel asks Loomis and Chunky for information on Ullmann, Lethem makes an unusual orthographical decision to italicize a word that does not resemble an interruptive tic: "Tell me *Ullmann's* address," I said for their sake. *Man-Salad-Dress* went my brain. I swallowed hard to keep it from crossing the threshold."[67] The italicization of the word "Ullmann" again marks it formally as a verbal tic embedded within an intentional statement, but the strangeness here lies in the fact that Lionel unintentionally tics the very word that he intended to say. As a result, Lionel's listeners remain potentially unaware of any change in his speech, and this masked tic then produces a mental stream of anagrammatism (the rewording of "Ullmann's address" into "Man-Salad-Dress") which Lionel manages to prevent from escaping his mouth.

The third and final type of verbal tic found in *Motherless Brooklyn* corresponds to the common folk-understanding of Tourette's in popular culture, namely, the sudden intrusion of offensive swear words or socially inappropriate remarks into regular conversation. In Lionel's case, these copralalic outbursts are relatively rare and are typically triggered directly by his environment or circumstances. When the boys discover that Frank's van has been vandalized, for example, Tony insists that "someone's sending a message," and Lionel's response is a more copralalic version of his riffing style of mimicry: "*'Fuckitmessage,'* I suggested impulsively."[68] During his conversation with the black homicide detective, Lionel is unable to avoid a more conventionally offensive outburst: "Can we go back to—*fuckmeblackcop*—back to talking nice now?"[69] Here Lethem's use of dashes and italics act to sanitize Lionel's racist copralalia, but the degree of his responsibility for these coprolalic moments is not always so clear-cut. After Frank's death, when the boys are debating how to handle the fact that the homicide detective knows where to find them, Lethem leaves the status of Lionel's cursing more ambiguous:

> "Fuck it," Coney said, "Fuck some fucking black cop."
> . . .
> "Fuckicide," I thought to add.[70]

One would expect a neologism like "fuckicide" to come from a tourettic outburst, but since it is not italicized, it would seem to be a voluntary statement. What makes this example even more ambiguous is the fact that it is quoted as dialogue, yet said to be something Lionel only "thought to add." Whether it was said aloud and whether it came from Lionel himself or from his tourettic self remain uncertain.

For the most part though, as I have shown, Lethem's orthographic decision has a stabilizing effect, leading us to wonder how different (and perhaps more interesting) a novel *Motherless Brooklyn* might be had Lethem chosen not to fix the difference between voluntary and involuntary utterances typographically.

At the same time, there are other counterexamples (similar to the perplexing arrangement of "fuckicide") that do not fit neatly into any of the three categories of verbal tics delineated above. These borderline cases are more difficult to interpret primarily because as readers we are led to expect ticcish language to be uniformly italicized. Early in the novel, Lethem offers a clue to the status of these borderline cases: "'Problyreallyoughttogo,' I said semicompulsively."[71] Here, the lack of italics works against the jamming together of the words into a ticcish style of delivery, signaling along with the adverb that this utterance is half-willed and half-unwilled. Interestingly, these unitalicized moments of ticcishness often coincide with Lionel's most creative utterances. One of the more comical instances of Lionel's straddling of the line between voluntary and involuntary utterance comes when he notices a cover story on the artist formerly known as Prince at a Casino newspaper stand. In 1993, Prince infamously changed his stage name to a popular glyph for Love that combines the symbols for male and female. In what can only be described as a primal act of originary language, Lionel finds himself groping to pronounce this unpronounceable glyph: "'Plavshk,' I said. My brain had decided to try to pronounce that unpronounceable glyph."[72] The result is a comic restaging of mankind's advance from hieroglyphic to alphabetic language, where Lionel goes on to test out several alternative pronunciations, each equally absurd. On the one hand, these coinages would appear to be tourettic speech since he tells us that his brain decides to pronounce the glyph in the first place, however, the word "plavshk" is not italicized, suggesting another act of creative wordplay performed "semicompulsively." Semicompulsiveness thus stands as the novel's model for understanding touretically creative wordplay. To put this in Kantian terms, these moments offer Lionel just the right amount of rule-governed freedom to experiment with language in truly creative ways.[73]

"Those walls of language"

While Lionel's own understanding of the cause of his disease is thoroughly neurological, it bears pointing out that Lethem has provided Lionel with an all-too-familiar backstory. He is an orphan, a child of motherless Brooklyn, and he finds a Mcmurphyesque father figure in Frank Minna, who both teases and encourages Lionel as a young boy. Although there is no permanent cure for his syndrome, Lionel constantly searches for ways to alleviate or mask his symptoms. During the initial eruption of his tics, Lionel tells us that he tries several medications—Haldol, Klonopin, and Orap—in the hopes of reducing his physical tics, but his attitude toward the side effects further situates him in the antipsychiatric tradition of Ken Kesey. "The chemicals slowed my brain to a morose crawl," Lionel explains, "I might outsmart my symptoms, disguise or incorporate them, frame them as eccentricities or vaudeville, but I wouldn't narcotize them, not if it meant dimming the world (or my brain—same thing) to twilight."[74] Here, the novel's neuromythological refrain—"the world (or my brain—same thing)"—does suggest that Lionel's experience of his world is ultimately reducible to the material workings of his brain, but the irony of his particular pathology is that it allows Lionel to hold onto a somewhat Humanist conviction that his tourettic brain is always "my *particular* brain" (emphasis added).[75] Lionel is for that very reason unwilling to "narcotize" his private, individualized world into a general darkness.[76] One of the ways that Lionel attempts to outsmart his physical tics is through speech itself. As the tic of all tics, language eventually supersedes his physical compulsions: "Speech, it turned out, liberated me from the overflowing disaster of my tourettic self, turned out to be the tic that satisfied where others didn't, the scratch that briefly stilled the itch."[77] Tourettic speech thus offers him an initial cure, although Lionel quickly realizes that speech can only briefly still his ticcishness and he is soon forced to disguise and modify his verbal tics the more humiliating they become.

The degree to which Lionel is able to achieve stillness quickly becomes his primary way of measuring how successful certain cures are for calming his twitchy compulsions. In line with the characters we examined in Chapter 3, Lionel discovers that one of the most effective means to achieve this stillness is sexual intercourse.[78] Although Lionel cannot be said to suffer the same level of sexual repression exhibited by Billy Bibbit, the isolating nature of Lionel's condition does limit his sexual contact with women. Lionel believes sexual activity directly diminishes the severity and frequency of his tourettic symptoms, an effect he describes in terms of a more focused stillness:

Sexual excitement stills my Tourette's brain, not by numbing me, dimming the world like Orap or Klonopin, those muffling medications, but instead by setting up a deeper attentiveness in me, a finer vibration, which gathers and encompasses my urgent chaos, enlists it in a greater cause, like a chorus of voices somehow drawing a shriek into harmony. I'm still myself and still in myself, a rare and precious combination.[79]

As in *Cuckoo's Nest* and *Temple of the Golden Pavilion*, sex in *Motherless Brooklyn* offers the Ticcer a temporary release from his symptoms, despite the fact that Tourette's and sexual repression are not troped by Lethem as interrelated forms of blockage. On the contrary, Lionel's syndrome produces an "urgent chaos," an excess of verbal and physical ejaculations. In a reverse way, then, sexual release enables Lionel not to unblock his speech but to block it, and by impeding his excesses, he is able to harmonize his two halves into a single "stilled self."[80]

Lionel's rare experiences of stillness can also be related to the issue of physical violence outlined in Chapters 3 and 4. Looking back to the case of Billy Budd, it is his inability to ejaculate verbally that compels him to physically ejaculate. Similarly for characters like Mizoguchi and Merry Levov, their psychic repression is so severe that they resort to physical destruction to alleviate their stutters. By contrast, the "urgent chaos" of Lionel's tourettic condition is such that only violence directed *at him* offers a temporary solution to his symptoms. The chaotic excess of Lionel's syndrome is held in check only when he is the target (not the instigator) of violence, for example, when Lionel is held at gunpoint by Tony, and feels "[his] ticcishness ease, and a flood of excess language instantly evaporate."[81] In fact, his condition only worsens when he resorts to violent actions, as when Lionel and Julia both hold each other at gunpoint late in the novel and Lionel notices that holding a gun triggers his ticcishness: "My syndrome had just discovered the prospect of the gun, and I began to obsess on pulling the trigger. I suspected that if I fired a shot out into the sky in the manner of my verbal exclamation, I might not survive the experience."[82] Here, Lionel links language, sexuality, and violence together in the same fashion of Melville's narrator, as interrelated forms of ejaculation. Resorting to violence only results in setting off new tics, and for Lionel, gunplay is ultimately only "another perfectly useless cure," even more short-lived than the benefits he reaps from sexual interplay.[83]

The failure to permanently cure his Tourette's through sexual activity is in part what leads Lionel to explore Zen meditation as another way of reducing his symptoms. Lethem's decision to incorporate Zen spirituality into the novel is particularly fitting since the emphasis in Zen meditation on physical and mental stillness stands in stark contrast to the uncontrollable ticcishness inherent in Tourette's syndrome. Kimmery explains to Lionel that Zen meditation is called *zazen*, or "*sitting*. It sounds like nothing, but it's the heart of Zen practice."[84] The practice of *zazen* involves regulating the mind and body by controlling one's endless stream of thoughts, allowing them to come and go without interference. By detaching from all levels of thought, the Zen meditator strives to contemplate nothing, thereby achieving what is sometimes called "One Mind."[85] This particular way of relating to one's body and mind would presumably sound completely foreign to a longtime sufferer of Tourette's like Lionel, whose ticcish condition is the polar opposite of the controlled stillness and silence of Zen sitting. At one point, Kimmery asks him, "What's wrong with you then?" to which he replies, "Nothing—at least from a Zen outlook."[86] The pun here on "nothing" implies that Lionel is unable to free his mind (or empty his brain) of intentional contents for the purpose of meditation. In short, the experience of Tourette's is a steady stream of "somethings," but the nothingness of Zen is the one something he has never been able to experience. In the novel's most comical juxtaposition of Zen and Tourette's, Lionel attempts to practice meditation with Kimmery, but while he is sitting, he can feel "all the more keenly the uneasy, half-stopped force of my own language-generator, my Multi-Mind, that tangle of responses and mimickings, of interruptions of interruptions."[87] He tries to unify and silence his mind, however, his tourettic brain constantly interrupts his concentration:

> The first thing I heard was Minna's voice: *I dare you to shut up for a whole twenty minutes sometime, you free human freakshow.*
> I pushed it away, thought *One Mind* instead.
> One Mind.
> *Tell me one, Freakshow. One I don't already know.*
> *I want to go to Tibet.*

One Mind. I focused my breathing.
Come home, Irving.
One Mind. Sick Mind. Dirty Mind. Bailey Mind.
One Mind.
Oreo Man.[88]

During this botched attempt at meditation, Lionel's tourettic stream-of-consciousness moves from mimicry to a consciously controlled focusing on the mantra of "One Mind," then back to mimicry, before shuttling off into a string of free associations. Much of the comedy of this scene comes from Lethem's stabilizing orthographics, with the tourettic brain interrupting Lionel's already fragile focus, while the other Lionel silently riffs on the Zen mantra in a futile attempt to detach himself from either of these cacophonous streams of thought. Lionel's comic failure to still his "Multi-mind" is so total that, while sitting on the floor beside Kimmery, he even begins to find himself sexually aroused by the thought of Kimmery's body. "As my penis stiffened," he tells us, "it occurred to me that I'd found my One Mind."[89]

The final proposed cure for Lionel's symptoms returns us to the question of environmental causes, and the effect on Lionel of living in a noisy, hectic modern city. Like Zola's Laurent, Lionel is overstimulated, or enervated, by New York. Moreover, like all inhabitants of the modern city, Lionel has little choice but to passively receive and process its many signs and signals, though his Tourette's for once actually makes him feel less alienated and more at home in this urban phantasmagoria than the average person. Lionel singles out the hotdog restaurant Papaya Czar as "my kind of place" due to the "bright orange and yellow signs pasted on every available surface screaming."[90] Through the synesthetic screaming of the restaurant walls, Lionel discovers another way in which his world and his brain are truly one and the same: "Papaya Czar's walls are so layered with language that I find myself immediately calmed inside their doors, as though I've stepped into a model interior of my own skull."[91] He makes an identical observation about the subway, where "the tunnel walls are layered, like those of my brain, with expulsive and incoherent language."[92] The relative calm Lionel feels at the hotdog shop, however, should not be mistaken as a source of relief for his Tourette's. The overabundance of signs in New York may make him feel at home or at one with his environment, but that feeling also exacerbates his tics. It is only when Lionel leaves the city, driving north toward Maine in pursuit of Tony, that he experiences an unexpected withdrawal of his symptoms:

> Waves, sky, trees, Essrog—I was off the page now, away from the grammar of skyscrapers and pavement. I experienced it precisely as a loss of language, a great sucking-away of the word-laden walls that I needed around me, that I touched everywhere, leaned on for support, cribbed from when I ticced aloud. Those walls of language had always been in place, I understood now, audible to me until the sky in Maine deafened them with a shout of silence. I staggered, put one hand on the rocks to steady myself. I needed to reply in some new tongue, to find a way to assert a self that had become tenuous.[93]

In this scene, Nature exists in opposition to the wordiness of the City, and when the walls of language are removed, Lionel finds himself suddenly, for the first time, at a loss for words. One of the ironies of this epiphanic moment is that Lionel is a self-described "*freak of nature*" whom only Nature can cure.[94] The sort of cure offered by Nature works less by stilling his brain than by starving it. The wordlessness of natural beauty provides his tourettic brain nothing to react to but pure silence, an obliteration of the Word, and his urge to tic is replaced with the search for a new tongue to assert his now wordless, ticless self. Lionel attempts to reclaim his "tenuous self" by shouting into the void:

> "Freakshow!" I yelled into the swirling foam. It was lost.
> "Bailey!" vanished too.
> "Eat me! Dickweed!"
> Nothing.[95]

With the urge to tic withdrawn, Lionel voluntarily tics aloud, almost testing the power of tourettic language against this wordless space. The result is the very goal his reactive self was unable to achieve through Zen meditation, the experience of Nothing.

"Tourette's muse was with me"

The complexity of tourettic language, with its inventive wordplay and incessant mutability, has led some critics to the tenuous conclusion that Tourette's syndrome is more than a mere disability, but rather a fundamentally creative and productive state of being. In his article "Tourette's Syndrome and Creativity," Oliver Sacks poses the question of whether artists with Tourette's, like Mozart or Samuel Johnson, were exceptional creators in spite of their syndrome, or whether their condition actually played an active role in their prolific careers. Sacks suggests that what he calls the "phantasmagoric form of Tourette's syndrome" possesses a transformative power to "touch, to interact with, a person's character and creativity and even to lend that person some of its own striking 'character.'"[96] In his article "The Poetics of Tourette's Syndrome," Ronald Schleifer builds on Sacks' argument by exploring the specific connections between tourettic speech and poetic language. Using Greimas' model of poetry as a "primal cry," Schleifer argues that the "uncanny verbalizations" of Tourette's syndrome not only resemble poetic language, but even function as a "source of much of poetry's power."[97] Schleifer points to Lionel's language in *Motherless Brooklyn* as one such example of the primordially poetic nature of tourettic speech, and it is certainly true that we often witness Lionel engaged in creatively poetic forms of wordplay. Across the many puns and neologisms, Lionel recognizes his brain's autonomous creative impulses: "It was as if my brain were inspired, trying to generate a really original new tic. Tourette's muse was with me."[98] If language in *Motherless Brooklyn* can be said to approach something like Greimas' primal cry, or the creative eruption of literary language suggested by Deleuze in his essay "He Stuttered," it is not a matter of the difference between voluntary and involuntary language in the novel, which as I have shown, is made stable by Lethem's orthographic decisions. A primal poetics within *Motherless Brooklyn* would have to come instead from the seemingly infinite tonal variations one finds in Lionel's ticced speech, which reach the same level of variation we located earlier in *Cuckoo's Nest*. Lionel's tics are vocalized alternately as abrupt screams, inaudible whispers, words muttered under the breath or between clenched teeth, sentences partially withheld and partially spoken.[99] Moreover, these tonal variations apply internally as well to the inner voice of Lionel's tourettic brain, which ranges from the loudest of shouts to the softest of murmurs. This polyphonic nature of language in *Motherless Brooklyn*, however, lends itself equally if not more so to novelistic discourse. The polyphony of voices competing to be heard within Lionel's

Multi-Mind bears striking similarities to Bakhtin's notion of the heteroglossic nature of novelistic discourse. In *The Dialogic Imagination*, Bakhtin sets the monoglossia of poetry in opposition to the heteroglossia of the Novel. For Bakhtin, the poet "accepts the idea of a unitary and singular language," and as such, the poet "strips the word of others' intentions."[100] By contrast, novelistic language is said to be "shot through with intentions and accents."[101] The novelistic word "becomes 'one's own' only when the speaker populates it with his own intention, his own accent, when he appropriates the word."[102] Not all words, however, submit equally to this act of appropriation. Many words, Bakhtin claims, "stubbornly resist, others remain alien, sound foreign in the mouth of the one who appropriated them."[103] Lionel's entire experience of language draws Bakhtin's insight out onto the surface of *Motherless Brooklyn*. As a tourettic narrator, Lionel is especially aware and uneasy about what it means to appropriate the words of others, and he experiences language as a pathological mixture of intentional and unintentional acts of appropriation: "Speech was intention, and I couldn't let anyone else know how intentional my craziness felt."[104] Perhaps the most complex and poignant experience of intention and appropriation comes at the novel's end, when Lionel meets with Kimmery for the last time and she informs him that she has decided to move back in with an old boyfriend:

> I opened my mouth and nothing came out.
> "You understand, Lionel?"
> "Ah." *Understand me, Bailey.*
> "Okay?"
> "*Okay*," I said. She didn't need to know it was just a tic, just echolalia that made me say it.
> "Okayokayokayokayokayokay" I said under my breath.[105]

Lionel's initial attempt to respond inverts his disordered speech into a kind of mutism, a prelinguistic state where no sound is made. When Kimmery asks if he understands, Lionel then progresses to the most primitive utterance possible, a monosyllabic open-vowelled sound. The vagueness of his answer prompts Kimmery to rephrase her question, and Lionel's answer reveals how appropriation for him so often means misappropriation. Even without Lionel's explanation that his reply is not voluntary but echolalic, the italicization of the "Okay" would delineate its status formally as another unintentional act of mimicry. What makes the scene so poignant is that Lionel allows this tic to disguise his real feelings and stand in for his true intention. In other words, Lionel chooses here to remain at the mercy of his syndrome, letting his ticced speech determine the final outcome of the situation. As if to will himself to mean what he says, Lionel then repeats the word several times, "Okayokayokayokayokayokay," in an unitalicized and more intentional whisper.

Since Lionel's "two disgruntled brains" exist in a constant struggle for dominance, language in the novel always consists like this of two speakers with two separate intentions. The overall result closely resembles what Bakhtin calls "double-voiced discourse" in which the character's speech and intentions are refracted by those of the author. For Bakhtin, these two dialogically related voices "know about each other, . . . it is as if they actually hold a conversation with each other."[106] With this in mind, a Bakhtinian approach to a novel like *Motherless Brooklyn* raises two interesting and difficult questions: first, about Lionel's status as a kind of unreliable narrator, in the limited sense that he is not fully in control of what he says, and second, about what it would mean for Lethem to be the implied author of a novel so shot through with intentionally unintentional utterances. In any case, if *Motherless Brooklyn* can be called a Bakhtinian text, this must be filtered through the central issue of speech pathology. The heteroglossia of *Motherless Brooklyn* is better described, therefore, as *hetero-glossolalia*, a pathologized version of the heteroglossic language to be found in all novels.

Conclusion: On Speech Disorders in Theory

"Song is not compatible with aphasia and a stuttering Amphion is an absurd figure indeed."

> – Paul de Man, "Anthropomorphism and Trope in the Lyric"

In the previous chapters, I have stressed the predominantly metaphorical purpose behind most literary representations of disordered speech. These conditions, when they appear in literary works at all, are consistently made to indicate something beyond themselves, whether about the personality of the character or about the nature of language itself. Where applicable, I have further shown the tendency for stigmas and stereotypes to attach themselves to these medical metaphors. Traits of nervousness and frailty, of sexual inexperience or impotence, and the channeling of these "defects" into sudden outbursts of violence—these are the hallmarks of most modern literary renderings of speech pathology. In this respect, modern literature has rarely sought to distance itself from what one critic has called the "coarse caricatures" to be found in more popular cultural forms such as film and television.[1] This dual process (of metaphor and stigma) has also led, as I have shown, to a proliferation of folk-etiologies and folk-remedies for these various conditions. In all of this, the treatment of speech disorders obeys a logic identical to the one elucidated by Susan Sontag in her work *Illness as Metaphor* (1978). According to Sontag, metaphorical associations (and subsequently moralistic judgments) are regularly projected onto different illnesses, however, since speech pathologies are neither terminal illnesses, nor even outwardly visible disabilities, they have traditionally occupied a marginal position at best in fields like the medical humanities and disability studies. In this work, I have tried to redress this marginalization by showing how those conditions that affect speech are no less prone to the kind of stigmatizing metaphorization described by Sontag. What she calls "punitive or sentimental fantasies" are regularly enacted through which broken speech is assigned a distinctly pejorative meaning as a sociocultural phenomenon.[2]

This tendency common to literary works—to make the basic fact of dysfluency meaningful beyond itself—can also be located in literary theory, but with a key difference that I will address briefly in this conclusion. Instead of judging speech disorders as evidence of some underlying characterological or linguistic defect, literary theorists more often take the exact opposite approach, glorifying or romanticizing forms of dysfluency as the manifestation of an idealized state of language. The most influential example of this approach comes in Gilles Deleuze's essay "He Stuttered," in which he offers a liberatory account of the creative potential in stuttering to "make a language take flight."[3] To underscore the purely metaphorical nature of what Deleuze is describing, it should be noted that with the practice he calls "creative stuttering," Deleuze insists the writer need not portray an actual act of stuttering at all.[4] This is because when it comes to creative stuttering, "it is no longer the character who stutters in speech; it is the writer who becomes *a stutterer in language*."[5] While Deleuze does briefly outline the two available ways of representing the actual speech-fluency disorder at the outset of his essay ("to do it" vs. "to say it without doing it"), his primary objective in "He Stuttered" is to elaborate a higher process through which certain writers by sheer force of style set standard language into a state of "perpetual disequilibrium."[6] The result is a situation where "the language itself will begin to vibrate and stutter, but without being confused with speech."[7] The role that actual stuttering plays in Deleuze's essay can only be described as a glorifying act of metaphor with no bearing on the lived experience of actual stutterers.

Deleuze is hardly alone among poststructuralist critics in adopting an idealizing attitude toward the breakdown of ordinary communicative speech. In this context, Michel de Certeau's essay "Vocal Utopias: Glossolalias" can also be singled out for its glorifying account of the specifically semantic form of breakdown known as glossolalia, or speaking in tongues. In his essay, de Certeau pushes toward a metaphorical form of glossolalia (again, outside its actual manifestation in religious contexts). This meta-glossolalia, much like

Deleuze's creative stuttering, is another disruptive force in this case generated within language itself, a force that "pushes up through the cracks of ordinary conversation."[8] For de Certeau, this vocal phenomenon belongs in the same category with other excessively nonstandard forms of language, including many of those I have examined throughout this work: "Literary, ludic, or infantile, and on occasion pathological, this form of glossolalia crosses through the boundary of statements to test the potentialities of the vocal palette."[9] The terminology de Certeau employs to describe the workings of this heightened state of language, a state which for him is always to some extent prelinguistic, probably comes closest to that used by Gail Jones in her novel *Sorry*. Like the character Perdita Keene, de Certeau's imagined glossolalic speaker seeks out a free space in which to play with vocalization, however, the sense of freedom here is not freedom from blockage but rather freedom from the shackles of meaning:

> As an invention of vocal space, glossolalia in fact multiplies the possibilities of speech. No determination of meaning constrains or restrains it. The decomposition of syllables and the combination of elementary sounds in games of alliteration create an *indefinite* space outside of the jurisdiction of a language.[10]

The idea implicit here that standard, fluent language confines us, and that the best liberation from this confinement comes through some amalgamation of literary and pathological forms began, of course, not with the poststructuralists, but with Russian formalists like Victor Shklovksy and Boris Eichenbaum. The social and literary forces to which these critics were responding are well known, but what is not usually noted is how often the Russian Formalists appropriated a vocabulary of speech pathology to describe the "defamiliarization" [*ostranenie*] of standard language that they espoused for modern literature. In 1923, for example, Eichenbaum wrote in reference to the Trans-sense poetry movement that, "it became necessary to create a new, *inarticulate, uncouth speech*, to emancipate the tradition of poetic diction from the shackles of Symbolism" (emphasis added).[11] Moreover, what characterized the new aesthetic of defamiliarization, for Shklovksy, was a "difficult, roughened, *impeded* language" (emphasis added).[12] In his seminal essay "Art as Technique," Shklovsky famously proposes that the defamiliarization of everyday language offers a certain corrective derangement through which both the significative powers of language and the perceptive capacities of the reader/listener are restored.

From the vantage point of this study, this uniquely modern viewpoint—that eloquence and fluency are the problem and dysfluency the solution—surely begs some rethinking. It should be asked why literary theory turns so consistently throughout the twentieth century to the realm of speech pathology to describe both the forms of literary experimentation and our culture's occasional need for language breakdown. It should also be asked whether it is possible to have a theoretical approach to disordered speech that is grounded in the more phenomenological aspects of language breakdown. A theory, in other words, that manages to avoid the many pitfalls I have laid out thus far, namely, metaphorization, stigmatization, and glorification. To avoid these pitfalls, one might be tempted simply to turn away from literary theory altogether toward more clinical approaches to these questions, such as can be found in emerging fields like Neurology of the Arts or Neuro-Lit-Crit. In my view, however, this is only to exchange one set of problems for another. Where the works of Deleuze and de Certeau prove overly metaphorical, offering us little by way of insight into actual disorders of speech, virtually all the work done in Neurology of the Arts proves overly reductive, offering us an impoverished account of the creative process and the meaning of the literary text. Work in this area by popularizers such as Oliver Sacks and Jonah Lehrer among others may at least provide a more rigorously clinical approach to the medical conditions in question, but as literary criticism, it rarely rises above the level of reductive platitudes and gross generalities.

It is not my intention here to argue against the value of interdisciplinarity as such when it comes to this topic, but rather to insist that the standard of interdisciplinarity for Neurology of the Arts needs to be higher. The appropriation of neurology and the fascination with neurological disorders so prevalent in contemporary literary and cultural theory needs to transcend the exploitative fascination of a Deleuze or the theoretical obfuscation of a Catherine Malabou. Likewise, those neurologists who endeavor to enter into literary criticism should respect the autonomous expertise of literary criticism and resist treating the literary object as though it existed merely to verify scientific hypotheses.[13] Throughout this work, I have attempted to practice the kind of rigorously interdisciplinary approach I am arguing for here. I have made my object of inquiry the literary texts themselves. I have avoided cracking open the brains of my authors, and though I have engaged in pathography at points where I believed it necessary to illuminate the literary works in question, I have never confused pathography of authors for actual literary criticism, as practitioners of Neurology of the Arts so often do. It is my hope that future work in this area will continue to avoid both metaphorization and reductionism, and that a form of criticism will develop which brings together literary criticism, neurology, and speech pathology into an authentically interdisciplinary understanding of the lived experience of speech pathology.

Notes

Introduction

1 See Macdonald Critchley, "Dr. Samuel Johnson's Aphasia," *Medical History* 6, 1 (January 1962): 27–44; and John Wiltshire, *Samuel Johnson in the Medical World: The Doctor and the Patient* (Cambridge: Cambridge University Press, 1991).

2 Critchley, "Letter 4, Chapman Collection," "Dr. Samuel Johnson's Aphasia," 30.

3 Howard Gardner, *The Shattered Mind: The Person After Brain Damage* (New York: Vintage, 1974), 89.

4 Critchley, "Letter 2, Chapman Collection," "Dr. Samuel Johnson's Aphasia," 29.

5 Critchley, "Letter 1, Chapman Collection," "Dr. Samuel Johnson's Aphasia," 29.

6 Charles Baudelaire, *Correspondance II (mars 1860-mars 1866)* (Paris: Gallimard, 1973), 397.

7 Julien Bogousslavsky and Sebastian Dieguez, "Baudelaire's Aphasia: From Poetry to Cursing," in *Neurological Disorders in Famous Artists, Part 2,* eds. Julien Bogousslavsky and Frantois Boller (New York: Karger, 2007), 129.

8 Charles Baudelaire, "L'aphasie." *Revue Neurologique* 125, 4 (1971), 129.

9 Charles Baudelaire, 26 March 1866 (my translation); See Bougollasavsky and Dieguez, and Lebrun et al. where appropriate: Bougollasavsky and Dieguez, "Baudelaire's Aphasia"; Yvan LeBrun, Janine Hasquin-Deleval, Jean Brihaye, and Jacques Flament, "L'aphasie de Charles Baudelaire." *Revue Neurologique* 125, 4 (October 1971): 310–16.

10 Paul Broca, *Ecrits sur l'aphasie (1861–1869)* (Paris: L'Harmattan, 2004), 111.

In 1859, Paul Broca founded the Paris Anthropological Society partly to protest the reception his work had received from the more ideologically conservative Societe de Biologie. In Broca's version of events, he was interrupted in the middle of a lecture by the biological society's president and was asked to withdraw his paper because of its clear overtones of polygenism (the view that the human race descends from multiple pairs), a dangerous position for scientists to hold during the reign of the fervently Catholic Second Empire. Indignant over this act of censorship, Broca formed the Societe d'Anthropologie de Paris that very night. In her study of nineteenth-century French anthropology, *The End of the Soul*, Jennifer Michael Hecht notes that "Broca's new society was thus controversial and defiant from its inception." Hecht, *The End of the Soul: Scientific Modernity, Atheism, and Anthropology in France* (New York: Columbia University Press, 2003), 56. Hecht situates Broca and his cohort in the generation of "freethinking anthropologists" whose scientific practices from the 1860s through the 1880s reflect the strong link between biological materialism and anticlerical atheism at that time. It is in this cultural climate that Broca's landmark case study is best understood, as one of the more visible examples of the threat that science then posed to both theist and humanist ideas about the true source of language.

11 Broca, *Ecrits sur l'aphasie*, 125.

12 Ibid., 104; 48.

13 Broca, *Ecrits sur l'aphasie*, 49; From English version in Paul Eling, ed., *Reader in the History of Aphasia* (Philadelphia: John Benjamins Publishing Company, 1994).

14 Broca, *Ecrits sur l'aphasie*, 109.

15 Broca, *Ecrits sur l'aphasie*, 111–2 (French); Broca in Eling, ed., *Reader in the History of Aphasia*, 41 (English).

16 L. S. Jacyna, *Lost Words: Narratives of Language and the Brain: 1825–1926* (Princeton, NJ: Princeton University, 2000). Originally published in Jean-Baptiste Bouillaud, *Archives Générales de Médicine* Paris 8 (1825): 30.

17 Broca, *Ecrits sur l'aphasie*, 121.

18 Ibid., 145.

19 Ibid., 142.

20 Broca, *Ecrits sur l'aphasie*, 142.

21 Ibid.

22 Ibid., 144.

23 Broca in Eling, ed., *Reader in the History of Aphasia*, 42.

24 Ibid.

25 Broca in Eling, ed., *Reader in the History of Aphasia*, 43 (English); Broca, *Ecrits sur l'aphasie*, 113 (French).

26 Broca also considered alogie, aphrasie. Note: Bastian as late as 1898 still distinguishes between aphemia (Broca's aphasia) and aphasia as two partly but not completely overlapping pathologies. Arthur L. Benton and Robert J. Joynt,

"Early Descriptions of Aphasia." *Archives of Neurology* 3 (1960), accessed 11 April 2010, http://www.archneurol.com.

27 Broca in Eling, ed., *Reader in the History of Aphasia*, 49.

28 Broca, *Écrits sur l'aphasie*, 138.

29 Critchley, "Letter 2, Chapman Collection," "Dr. Samuel Johnson's Aphasia," 29; "Letter 3, Chapman Collection," 29; and see Axel Karenberg, "Cerebral Localisation in the Eighteenth Century – An Overview." *Journal of the History of the Neurosciences* 18 (2009): 248–53.

30 James Boswell, *Life of Johnson: Unabridged* (Oxford: Oxford University Press, 1998), 1224.

31 Ibid., 1225.

32 Critchley, "Letter 4, Chapman Collection," "Dr. Samuel Johnson's Aphasia," 3.

33 Critchley, "Letter 2, Chapman Collection," "Dr. Samuel Johnson's Aphasia," 29.

34 Critchley, "Letter 8, Chapman Collection," "Dr. Samuel Johnson's Aphasia," 32.

35 Although Johnson did note his writing difficulties, he seems never to have made the connection between his agraphia and his aphasia. "My hand," he wrote about his initial letter to Edmund Allen, "I knew not how nor why, made wrong letters." The basic aphasiological premise that these two difficulties shared the same cause (damage to the language center itself) seems to have escaped him.

36 Critchley, "Letter 12, Chapman Collection," "Dr. Samuel Johnson's Aphasia," 33.

37 In the past 50 years, aphasiologists have attempted to perform posthumous "case studies" of the strokes and subsequent aphasias of both Samuel Johnson and Charles Baudelaire, without the benefit of postmortem autopsy, basing their findings on the available pathographical evidence. In his 1960 study, "Dr. Samuel Johnson's Aphasia," Macdonald Critchley compiled the various reports from Johnson's own letters and those of his friends and doctors. He concluded that the mildness of the aphasia in this case, along with the almost total lack of facial or other motor paralysis, indicates a lesion "small in size, and ischemic rather than thrombotic or haemorrhagic in nature." Critchley, "Dr. Samuel Johnson's Aphasia," 27–44. Two similar studies have been conducted on the case of Baudelaire. The first, entitled "L'aphasie de Charles Baudelaire," was published in the *Revue Neurologique* in 1971 by four neurologists from Brussels, Lebrun et al., "L'aphasie de Charles Baudelaire," 310–16. In 2007, Sebastian Dieguez and Julien Bogousslavsky of the Brain Mind Institute in Lausanne published a study building on the work of Lebrun: Bogousslavsky and Dieguez, "Baudelaire's Aphasia: From Poetry to Cursing."

38 Bogousslavsky and Dieguez, "Baudelaire's Aphasia: From Poetry to Cursing," 130.

39 Samuel Johnson, *A Dictionary of the English Language: An Anthology* (London: Penguin Books, 2005), 24.

40 Baudelaire, "L'aphasie," 313. Originally published in J. Crépet, "Les derniers jours de Charles Baudelaire." *La Nouvelle Revue Française* 21 (1932): 641–71.

41 Baudelaire, Correspondence Vol. 2, p. 629.

Chapter 1

1 See Jacyna, *Lost Words*, 118; Originally an intern in medicine and surgery at the Hopitaux de Paris, and briefly a student of Charcot's in 1883, Bernard was appointed as a professor of pathology and clinical surgery at the medical school in Marseille on the basis of his thesis *De L'aphasie* which he submitted to the Faculte de Paris, on the basis of which he was appointed as a professor of pathology and surgery at the medical school in Marseille, shortly after which Bernard died of a sudden illness before its publication in 1889. The diverse forms of aphasia which Bernard set out to clarify in his monograph were those conditions that affect how words are "heard and articulated, read, and fixed in writing," that is, word-deafness, aphemia, word-blindness, and agraphia, respectively. Désiré Bernard, *De L'Aphasie et De Ses Diverses Formes* (Paris: Publications du Progrès Médical, Par Ch. Féré, Médicin de Bicêtre, 1889), 264.

2 Bernard, *De L'Aphasie et De Ses Diverses Formes*, 7 (my translation).

3 Ibid., 8–9 (my translation).

4 Jacyna, *Lost Words*, 117.

5 Émile Zola, *Thérèse Raquin* (London: Penguin Books, 1962), 200.

6 Isabelle Delamotte, "La place de Charcot dans la documentation médicale d'Émile Zola." *Cahiers Naturalistes* 73 (1999).

7 "La paralysie gagnait peu à peu madame Raquin, et ils prévirent le jour où elle serait clouée dans son fauteuil, impotente et hébétée. La pauvre vieille commençait à balbutier des lambeaux de phrases qui se cousaient mal les uns aux autres; sa voix faiblissait, ses membres se mouraient un à un." Émile Zola, *Thérèse Raquin* (Paris: Garnier-Flammarion, 1970), 187.

8 Zola, *Thérèse Raquin* (London: Penguin Books, 1962), 199 (English); Zola, *Thérèse Raquin*, (Paris: Garnier-Flammarion, 1970), 206 (French).

9   Zola, *Thérèse Raquin* (London: Penguin Books, 1962), 204 (English); Zola, *Thérèse Raquin* (Paris: Garnier-Flammarion, 1970), 210 (French).

10 Zola, *Thérèse Raquin* (London: Penguin Books, 1962), 205; 210 (English); Zola, *Thérèse Raquin* (Paris: Garnier-Flammarion, 1970), 206; 215(French).

11 The absence of any of the accompanying symptoms of agraphia or alexia that might be expected in a case of aphasia adds weight to the argument that Madame's case does not quite reflect a post-1861 sense of language loss. Following the paralysis of her speech organs, "for a few days, Madame Raquin kept the use of her hands and could write on a slate and ask for what she wanted; but then her hands went dead too." Zola, *Thérèse Raquin* (London: Penguin Books, 1962), 201. Madame Raquin does momentarily regain her ability to write in that pivotal scene when she tries to expose Laurent and Thérèse as the murderers of her son. Appealing to her dinner guests, Michaud, Grivet and Olivier, the stricken woman desperately traces letters on the table with her finger: "Knowing that her tongue was quite dead she tried a new language. With an amazing effort of will she managed to force a little life back into her right hand and . . . feebly moved her fingers as if to attract attention." Zola, *Thérèse Raquin* (London: Penguin Books, 1962), 210. With this "new language," Madame Raquin's hand replaces her tongue as the instrument of communication. Making no mistakes, she traces out the partial phrase, "Thérèse and Laurent have . . . ." Before she is able to finish the sentence, however, "her fingers had stiffened, the supreme effort of will that had animated them was dying, and she could feel the paralysis creeping down her arm." Zola, *Thérèse Raquin* (London: Penguin Books, 1962). Although Madame's intelligence is not shown to be affected, there is no indication here or elsewhere that the specific faculty of language has been affected, nor even that the faculties of speech and of language are being distinguished from one another.

12 David F. Bell, "Thérèse Raquin: Scientific Realism in Zola's Laboratory." *Nineteenth Century French Studies* 24 (1995 Fall to 1996 Winter): 122–32; Isabelle Delamotte, "La place de Charcot dans la documentation médicale d'Émile Zola." *Cahiers Naturalistes* 73 (1999): 287–99; Henri Mitterand, ed., Introduction to *Oeuvres completes* by Émile Zola (*Thérèse Raquin* in Vol.1) (Paris: Cercle du Livre Précieux, 1960-7); Lilian R. Furst, "A Question of Choice in the Naturalistic Novel: Zola's *Thérèse Raquin* and Dreiser's *An American Tragedy*," in Proceedings of the Comparative Literature Symposium

(Lubbock: The Texas Tech Press, 1972), 39–53; Andrew Rothwell, Introduction to *Thérèse Raquin* by Émile Zola (Oxford: Oxford University Press World's Classics, 1992).

13　Zola, *Thérèse Raquin* (London: Penguin Books, 1962), 22.

14　Ibid.

15　Mitterand, ed., Introduction to *Oeuvres completes* by Émile Zola (*Thérèse Raquin* in Vol. 1), 18.

16　Benton and Joynt, "Early Descriptions of Aphasia," 207.

17　Pierre Larousse, *Grand dictionnaire universel du XIXe siècle* (Paris: Larousse et Boyer, 1865–90).

18　Larousse, *Grand dictionnaire*.

19　Zola, *Thérèse Raquin* (London: Penguin Books, 1962), 222 (English); Zola, *Thérèse Raquin*, (Paris: Garnier-Flammarion, 1970), 226 (French).

20　Zola, *Thérèse Raquin* (London: Penguin Books, 1962), 248; 214 (English – my translations); 171; Zola, *Thérèse Raquin* (Paris: Garnier-Flammarion, 1970), 246; 219; 182 (French).

21　Zola, *Thérèse Raquin* (London: Penguin Books, 1962), 188 (English); Zola, *Thérèse Raquin* (Paris: Garnier-Flammarion, 1970), 198 (French).

22　Zola, *Thérèse Raquin* (London: Penguin Books, 1962), 41.

23　Ibid., 39.

24　Ibid., 39; 63.

25　Ibid., 53.

26　Zola, *Thérèse Raquin* (London: Penguin Books, 1962), 22. Several critics have questioned the effectiveness of Zola's method in *Thérèse Raquin* either by deeming the "science" behind his method pseudo-scientific or by questioning the possibility for readers of the novel to do what the narration asks of them, that is, interpret characters neurophysiologically. The most persuasive argument against the workability of Zola's method is made by Lilian Furst, in her comparative study of Theodore Dreiser's *An American Tragedy* and Zola's *Thérèse Raquin*. See Furst, "A Question of Choice in the Naturalistic Novel: Zola's *Thérèse Raquin* and Dreiser's *An American Tragedy*." Furst claims that, "the reader inevitably 'translates' all this physiology and chemistry back into the emotive vocabulary usually associated with human relationships. We think of Thérèse's and Laurent's loves and hates, of their guilt and remorse rather than of their cerebral disorders." Furst, "A Question of Choice in the Naturalistic Novel," 52. Rothwell, in his Introduction to Zola's *Thérèse Raquin*, has similarly noted

that the absence of any ethical considerations makes it difficult to sympathize
with or condemn the couple: "Zola works hard to deny the reader two key
privileges which centuries of increasingly refined psychological literature had
accustomed him or her to enjoying as of right: those of identifying with the
characters' motives and feelings, and of judging their actions." Andrew Rothwell,
Introduction, viii.

27 Zola, *Thérèse Raquin* (London: Penguin Books, 1962), 114 (English); Zola,
Thérèse Raquin (Paris: Garnier-Flammarion, 1970), 127 (French).

28 Zola, *Thérèse Raquin* (London: Penguin Books, 1962), 84 (English); Zola,
Thérèse Raquin (Paris: Garnier-Flammarion, 1970), 110 (French).

Note – I have slightly altered the available English translations because
in almost every case, they make a key mistake translating "leur cerveau" as
plural instead of singular. Obviously for the purposes of the neurological
argument that I am making about Zola, it is important to note that *Thérèse* and
Laurent are said to share a single brain.

29 Zola, *Thérèse Raquin* (London: Penguin Books, 1962), 170 (English); Zola,
Thérèse Raquin (Paris: Garnier-Flammarion, 1970), 182 (French).

30 Claude Bernard, *An Introduction to the Study of Experimental Medicine*
(New York: The Macmillan Company, 1927), 88 (English); Claude Bernard,
Introduction à l'étude de la médicine expérimentale (Paris: Flammarion, 1952),
134 (French).

31 Zola, *Thérèse Raquin* (London: Penguin Books, 1962), 170.

32 Ibid., 171; 172.

33 Ibid., 172.

34 Zola, *Thérèse Raquin* (London: Penguin Books, 1962), 171 (English); Zola,
Thérèse Raquin (Paris: Garnier-Flammarion, 1970), 183 (French).

One of the few comic elements of *Thérèse Raquin* develops out of this study
of the mixing of sanguine and nervous temperaments. Zola seems to poke fun
at the cliché of the artist as a peasant who comes to the city by having Laurent
turn temporarily into an artist. He acquires a "feminine nervous system" and
the "quasi-moral disease or neurosis which had disturbed his whole being had
developed in him a strangely lurid artistic sense." Zola, *Thérèse Raquin* (London:
Penguin Books, 1962), 195.

35 In "Medicine and the Case of Emile Zola," Garabed Eknoyan and Byron A.
Eknoyan provide an incomplete catalogue of various diseases that appear in
the works of Zola, including smallpox, alcoholism, peritonsilar abscess, sepsis,

dementia, phenylketonuria, congestive heart failure, gout, anthracosis, and cerebrovascular accident (or stroke). Virtually all of Zola's novels foreground some form of disease, whether common afflictions like smallpox (*Nana*), dementia (*Docteur Pascal*), gout (*La Joie de Vivre*), sepsis (*La Débacle*), or heart failure (*La Joie de Vivre*), or more exotic conditions like anthracosis (*Germinal*) and phenylketonuira (*Docteur Pascal*). As an example of cerebrovascular accident in Zola, they do not list the case of Madame Raquin but rather the case of Fouan in *La Terre*. Other examples of apoplexy in Zola's corpus include *La faute de l'Abbét Mouret*, when Doctor Pascal goes to check on Old Jeanbernat "who had had an apoplectic stroke," only to find the old man has already bled himself and recovered. Émile Zola, *La faute de l'Abbé Mouret* (New York: Mondial, 2005), 30. Uncle Gradelle, the proprietor of the charcuterie in *Le Ventre de Paris*, dies suddenly one morning, "struck down by a stroke while preparing a *galantine*." Émile Zola, *The Belly of Paris* [*Le Ventre de Paris*] (New York: Oxford University Press, 2009), 47. Numerous other minor characters like the Prince d'Orviedo (*L'argent*), Monsieur Vabre (*Pot-Bouille*), and Deslignieres (*Au Bonheur des Dames*) all suffer attacks of apoplexy, and the mine-owner Deneulin from *Germinal*, when he finds himself facing financial collapse, "hoped he would die of a rush of blood to the head, choked by apoplexy." Émile Zola, *Germinal* (London: Penguin Books, 2004), 385.

36 Émile Zola, *The Earth* (London: Elek, 1967), 41.

37 Zola, *The Earth* (London: Elek, 1967), 335; 336.

38 Zola, *The Earth* (London: Elek, 1967), 90 (English); Zola, *La Terre* (Paris: Cercle du live précieux, 1969), 103 (French).

39 Zola, *The Earth* (London: Elek, 1967), 91 (English); Zola, *La Terre* (Paris: Cercle du live précieux, 1969), 104 (French).

40 Zola, *The Earth* (London: Elek, 1967), 91.

41 Rothwell, Introduction, xxi.

42 Zola, *Thérèse Raquin* (London: Penguin Books, 1962), 199 (English – my translation); Zola, *Thérèse Raquin* (Paris: Garnier-Flammarion, 1970), 206 (French).

43 Jacyna, *Lost Words*, 119.

44 Zola, *Thérèse Raquin* (London: Penguin Books, 1962), 202 (English); Zola, *Thérèse Raquin* (Paris: Garnier-Flammarion, 1970), 208 (French).

45 Zola, *Thérèse Raquin* (London: Penguin Books, 1962), 232.

46 Ibid., 240.

47 Zola, *Thérèse Raquin* (London: Penguin Books, 1962), 240 (English); Zola, *Thérèse Raquin* (Paris: Garnier-Flammarion, 1970), 240 (French).

48 Zola, *Thérèse Raquin* (London: Penguin Books, 1962), 240.

49 While the tale of Madame Raquin does not offer the fully accurate portrayal of the Aphasic with which Désiré Bernard credits the young Zola, Zola's depiction of Madame as a "walled-in intelligence" does reflect a post-Broca sensibility in one crucial respect. Zola, *Thérèse Raquin* (London: Penguin Books, 1962), 246. The brief access to her interiority tells us that Madame has not suffered from any diminished intelligence, which corresponds with Broca's conviction that individuals with aphemia still "hear and understand everything that is said to them." Broca in Eling, ed., *Reader in the History of Aphasia*, 43. Similarly, we are told that Madame Raquin "could see, hear, and reason in a clear and sensible way," and in this sense, it does seem to be that only her ability to articulate words which has been affected. Zola, *Thérèse Raquin* (London: Penguin Books, 1962), 273. In direct contrast to Madame's inability to communicate her thoughts to others, Thérèse's and Laurent's status as a single organism allows them to communicate without speaking at all, to read each other's minds through a "sorte de divination." Zola, *Thérèse Raquin* (London: Penguin Books, 1962), 193. Their crime binds them together so intimately that they "conversed, heart to heart and with no need for words, while talking about something else. Without even being conscious of the words they were saying, they followed out their secret thoughts sentence by sentence, and if they had suddenly gone aloud, the thread of their understanding would not have been broken." Zola, *Thérèse Raquin* (London: Penguin Books, 1962), 162. Though their spoken words rarely reflect their internal thoughts, they possess a mutual understanding that has "no need for words," signifying an organic synthesis so complete that conversation becomes unnecessary, even meaningless. But this seamless albeit silent form of communication becomes so unbearable to them that when Madame suffers her stroke, they use her to break up the ceaseless transfer of thoughts between them. It is only when Madame inadvertently uncovers the secret that Thérèse and Laurent have murdered her son that access to her interiority is briefly restored. Her private experience of language loss is rendered most clearly in the dinner scene already discussed where Madame attempts to communicate with her hand in an effort to expose the crime to her guests. Only the family friend Grivet tries to access her "walled-in intelligence," assuming that he and Madame

share something like the wordless communication of Thérèse and Laurent, a "complete sympathy . . . that she only had to glance at him and he grasped her meaning instantly." Zola, *Thérèse Raquin* (London: Penguin Books, 1962), 202. When Madame Raquin finds herself unable to finish writing her message, Grivet brags that he alone can read Madame's eyes and incorrectly guesses at what she wants to say: "She wanted to say: 'Thérèse and Laurent have been very good to me." Zola, *Thérèse Raquin* (London: Penguin Books, 1962), 213.

50 Marcel Proust, *Correspondance générale* (Paris: Plon, 1970–73), 5: 342.

51 Marcel Proust, *Remembrance of Things Past*, 3 vols (New York: Vintage Books, 1982), II: 344.

52 Marcel Proust, *Remembrance of Things Past*, 3 vols (New York: Vintage Books, 1982), II: 346 (English); Marcel Proust, *A la recherche du temps perdu*, 4 vols (Paris: Bibliothèque de la Pléiade, 1988), II: 630 (French).

53 Marcel Proust, *Essais et articles, presentation de Thierry Laget* (Paris: Éditions Gallimard, 1994), 317.

54 Julien Bogousslavsky, "Marcel Proust's Diseases and Doctors: The Neurological Story of a Life," in Julien Bogousslavsky and Frantois Boller (eds), *Neurological Disorders in Famous Artists, Part 2* (New York: Karger, 2007), 98.

55 Marcel Proust, *Remembrance of Things Past*, 3 vols (New York: Vintage Books, 1982), II: 336.

56 Marcel Proust, *Remembrance of Things Past*, 3 vols (New York: Vintage Books, 1982), II: 337 (English); Marcel Proust, *A la recherche du temps perdu*, 4 vols (Paris: Bibliothèque de la Pléiade, 1988), II: 621 (French).

It is worth noting here the exact term that Proust uses to describe Bergotte's speech troubles, since it is the very same term that is applied to Marcel's grandmother. Both cases are described as an "embarras de la parole," which when used reflexively, denotes not embarrassment but the experience of a burden.

57 In *The Guermantes Way*, Brissaud's fictional surrogate is described as "a specialist in nervous diseases, the man to whom Charcot before his death had predicted that he would reign supreme in neurology and psychiatry," but interestingly, in *Sodom and Gomorrah II*, Doctor Cottard makes a disparaging reference to Du Boulbon's less conventional methods as "a sort of literary medicine." Marcel Proust, *Remembrance of Things Past*, 3 vols (New York: Vintage Books, 1982), II: 311 (English); Marcel Proust, *A la recherche du temps perdu*, 4 vols (Paris: Bibliothèque de la Pléiade, 1988), II: 1009 (French).

58 Julien Bogousslavsky, "Marcel Proust's Lifelong Tour of the Parisian
    Neurological Intelligentsia: From Brissaud and Dejerine to Sollier and Babinski."
    European Neurology 57 (January 2007): 132.

59 Bogousslavsky, "Marcel Proust's Lifelong Tour of the Parisian Neurological
    Intelligentsia," 131.

60 Céleste Albaret, *Monsieur Proust* (Paris: Robert Laffont, 1973), 352.

61 Adrien Proust, *L'Aphasie* (Paris: Libraire de la Faculté de Médicine, Place de
    l'Ecole-de-Médicine, 1872), 26.

62 Adrien Proust, *L'Aphasie*, 5.

63 One of the more overtly Proustian digressions is a remark Adrien Proust makes
    about artists: "The gap between an ordinary man and a great man over the
    course of their lives is often almost imperceptible, while at the same time, being
    vast. An untalented painter can conceive the idea for a painting as perfect as
    those painted by Raphael, but when the moment of execution arrives, his brush
    refuses to transfer his ideas. A writerly hack conceives the layout for a dramatic
    work, but when he goes to fill the canvas, the means fail him." Adrien Proust,
    L'Aphasie, 15.

64 Adrien Proust, *L'Aphasie*, 7–8.

65 Ibid., 8.

66 Adrien Proust, *L'Aphasie*, 9. All of these reflections on the nature of language
    itself are a perfect example of a point George Steiner makes in his book
    After Babel. In the context of aphasiology, Steiner reminds us that, "virtually
    everything we know of the organization of the functions of language in the
    human brain derives from pathology. George Steiner, *After Babel: Aspects of
    Language and Translation* (Oxford: Oxford University Press, 1992), 282. In the
    same sense here, we find Dr Proust working backwards from a symptom of
    language breakdown to an understanding of what language is.

67 Adrien Proust, *L'Aphasie*, 23 (my translation).

68 Jacyna, *Lost Words*, 83.

69 Carl Wernicke, *Wernicke's Works on Aphasia: A Sourcebook and Review,*
    ed. Gertrude H. Eggert (The Hague: Mouton Publishers, 1977), 103.

70 Wernicke, *Works on Aphasia*, 121.

71 Two years prior to the publication of Wernicke's ten case studies in *The Aphasia
    Symptom-Complex*, Dr Proust in his *L'aphasie* seems almost to anticipate the
    copious (or "fluent") form of sensory aphasia that would soon be named after
    Wernicke, for instance, with the case of his patient number 19, known as

Clara X. When Dr Proust asked Clara to recite from a text she'd never seen before, she produced, in his words a "mixture of meaningless sounds" ["un mélange de sons sans signification"]. When he then asked her to write him a letter, the result was one of the earliest recorded cases of the condition now known as neologistic jargonaphasia: "Je suis tére de rampere campere, ailzanne, anise dans reste donc tres et sant et dont manssaa daupère et dans sanpaire ont d'aimumpè et sansces, dans d'austre d'oustre." Adrien Proust, *L'Aphasie*, 20.

72 Wernicke, *Wernicke's Works on Aphasia*, 108.

73 Ibid., 119.

74 Jacyna, *Lost Words*, 195.

75 These were exactly the kinds of questions Broca (who died in 1880) would have hoped his life's work would elicit. In her study of nineteenth-century French anthropology, *The End of the Soul*, Jennifer Michael Hecht situates Broca and his followers in the generation of "freethinking anthropologists" whose scientific practices from the 1860s through the 1880s reflect the strong link between biological materialism and anticlerical atheism at that time. In 1859, Paul Broca founded his Paris Anthropological Society partly to protest the reception his work had received from the more ideologically conservative Societe de Biologie. In Broca's version of events, he was interrupted in the middle of a lecture by the biological society's president and asked to withdraw his paper because of its clear overtones of polygenism (the view that the human race descends from multiple pairs), a dangerous position for scientists to hold during the reign of the fervently Catholic Second Empire. Indignant over this act of censorship, Broca formed the Societe d'Anthropologie de Paris that very night. Hecht notes that "Broca's new society was thus controversial and defiant from its inception." Hecht, *The End of the Soul*, 56. It is in this cultural climate that the development of aphasiology is best understood, as one of the more visible examples of the threat that positivist science posed in the late nineteenth century to both theist and humanist ideas about the true source of language.

76 Jacyna, *Lost Words*, see chapter 6.

77 In the Introduction to *On Aphasia*, E. Stengel notes that several key psychoanalytic concepts are already prefigured in this early text. "The speech apparatus," writes Stengel, "is the elder brother of the "psychic apparatus" to the working of which most of Freud's later researches were devoted."
E. Stengel, Introduction to *On Aphasia: A Critical Study* by Sigmund Freud. New York: International Universities Press, Inc., 1953, xiii. Stengel notes that

the theory of regression also finds its first articulation in *On Aphasia*, during Freud's discussion of marginally diminished states of language as "instances of functional retrogression (disinvolution) of a highly of a highly organized apparatus." Stengel, Introduction, xii.

78 Sigmund Freud, *On Aphasia: A Critical Study* (New York: International Universities Press, Inc., 1953), 105. Five years later in *Matter and Memory*, Bergson would make an almost identical comment: "The complication of the theories of aphasia being thus self-destructive, it is no wonder that modern pathology, becoming more and more skeptical with regard to diagrams, is returning purely and simply to the description of facts." Henri Bergson, *Matter and Memory* (New York: Dover Publications Inc., 2004), 158.

79 Freud, *On Aphasia*, 13.

80 Sigmund Freud, *Psychopathology of Everyday Life*, in *The Basic Writings of Sigmund Freud*, ed. and trans. Dr A. A. Brill (New York: The Modern Library, 1995), 5.

81 Freud, *Psychopathology of Everyday Life*, 18.

82 Ibid.

83 Ibid., 49.

84 Ibid., 54.

85 Marcel Proust, *Remembrance of Things Past*, 3 vols (New York: Vintage Books, 1982), III.895.

86 Ibid., III.893.

87 Ibid., III.895.

88 Marcel Proust, *Remembrance of Things Past*, 3 vols (New York: Vintage Books, 1982), III.893 (English); Marcel Proust, *A la recherche du temps perdu*, 4 vols (Paris: Bibliothèque de la Pléiade, 1988), IV.440 (French).

89 It should also be pointed out here that the technical term "progressive aphasia" does not appear in the French text. In the original version, Charlus is said to complain "qu'il allait a l'aphasie," that is, he says literally that he has *been going through* aphasia. The use of the imperfect tense here gives the description an idiomatic sense of aphasia as a persistent and worsening state that Charlus has been undergoing for some time. Marcel Proust, *A la recherche du temps perdu*, 4 vols (Paris: Bibliothèque de la Pléiade, 1988), IV.440.

90 Marcel Proust, *Remembrance of Things Past*, 3 vols (New York: Vintage Books, 1982), III.892.

91 Ibid., III.893.

92 Ibid., III.894.

93 Freud, *On Aphasia*, 13.

94 Marcel Proust, *Remembrance of Things Past*, 3 vols (New York: Vintage Books, 1982), III.209.

95 Ibid., III.206–7.

96 Ibid., III.209.

97 Marcel Proust, *Remembrance of Things Past*, 3 vols (New York: Vintage Books, 1982), III.321 (English); Marcel Proust, *A la recherche du temps perdu*, 4 vols (Paris: Bibliothèque de la Pléiade, 1988), III.820 (French).

98 Marcel Proust, *Remembrance of Things Past*, 3 vols (New York: Vintage Books, 1982), III.820.

99 Marcel Proust, *Remembrance of Things Past*, 3 vols (New York: Vintage Books, 1982), III.322 (English); Marcel Proust, *A la recherche du temps perdu*, 4 vols (Paris: Bibliothèque de la Pléiade, 1988), III.821 (French).

100 Marcel Proust, *Remembrance of Things Past*, 3 vols (New York: Vintage Books, 1982), III.221.

101 Gérard Genette, *Figures II* (Paris: Éditions du Seuil, 1969), 223.

102 Genette, *Figures II*, 223 (my translation).

103 Marcel Proust, *Remembrance of Things Past*, 3 vols (New York: Vintage Books, 1982), II.819.

104 Ibid., III.738.

105 Ibid.

Chapter 2

1 The war historian Sophie Delaporte estimates in *Gueules Cassées de la Grande Guerre* [*The Shattered Faces of the Great War*] that somewhere between 11 per cent and 14 per cent of French injured soldiers were wounded in the head or face. Of the 2,800,000 French wounded soldiers, that would amount to between 28,000 and 39,000 soldiers. Of these head and facial wounds, Delaporte estimates that 10,000–15,000 would have been deemed serious injuries. From the available statistics, we can only attempt to surmise the number of cases of disordered speech which these wounds would have caused, whether from damage to the brain or to the vocal organs. It is certain that World War I brought a new level of public visibility to these related conditions.

Sophie Delaporte, *Gueules Cassées de la Grande Guerre* [*The Shattered Faces of the Great War*] (Paris: Broché Épuisé, 2004).

2 Henry Head, *Aphasia and Kindred Disorders of Speech: In Two Volumes* (New York; London: Hafner Publishing Company, 1963), I.146.

3 While these case studies offer a novel glimpse into the horrors of the War and the struggles of the aphasic soldier long afterward, Head's tone throughout is unexpectedly optimistic about the benefits for science of access to this new type of patient. Head even points out the relative "advantage" of bullet wounds over the type of lesions caused by stroke: "With gun-shot wounds of the head the symptoms tend to clear up to a considerable extent, provided there are no secondary complications, even though the effect produced by the initial impact of the bullet may have been extremely severe. Some aspects of the disordered functions of speech recover more rapidly than others and the clinical manifestations assume more or less characteristic forms. In the end the patient may recover his powers to such an extent that he no longer fails to carry out the rough and simple tests which can be employed in clinical research; or on the other hand some aptitude may remain permanently defective. By this means we are enabled to trace the various steps by which the defective functions are restored, whereas in civilian practice any change in the clinical manifestations is usually in an opposite direction. Even if the vascular lesion is stationary, the symptoms rarely disappear, while in most cases the condition of the patient gradually deteriotates." Head, *Aphasia and Kindred Disorders of Speech*, I.146.

4 Head, *Aphasia and Kindred Disorders of Speech*, II.x.

5 Jacyna, *Lost Words*, See Chapter 5 "Head Wounds" for a fuller discussion of Henry Head's role in the development of the aphasiological case study.

6 Head, *Aphasia and Kindred Disorders of Speech*, II.x.

7 Ibid., II.89–107.

8 Another characteristic case is Patient number 1, a 22-year-old lieutenant and a former student of classics who was placed under Head's care at the London Hospital in November 1915. One month before, Patient #1 had suffered a shrapnel wound in a trench and undergone surgery. When Head conducted his first interview of the lieutenant, "he was completely speechless except for "yes" and "no" .... Articulation was extremely bad and he could not repeat even single words with certainty. He failed to understand what was said to him and executed oral commands with difficulty." Head, *Aphasia and Kindred Disorders of Speech*, II.1. After 30 weeks, however, Head reports that Patient #1 "had now

regained his old intellectual vigor. He was bright, cheerful, and in no way cast down by his disabilities." With respect to language, he now "talked slowly and with obvious difficulty . . . . He understood all that was said and executed even complex oral commands correctly." Head, *Aphasia and Kindred Disorders of Speech*, II.10, 1.

9 Jacyna, *Lost Words*, 152. In the section of Jacyna's chapter on Henry Head entitled "Finding the Ideal Patient," Jacyna also points out traces of classism in Head's implementation of his methodology. Head returns again and again throughout the case studies to the issue of the education level and intelligence of the patient, because the primary obstacle for the aphasic case study is gauging how the patient would have responded to the various speaking and writing tests prior to their head wound. One of the cornerstones of Head's individualizing approach was to trust the individual patient to assess their own prior capacities against their current impairments. But as Jacyna shows, there are hints that Head's trust in his patients to do so depended on their education and background: "Head was able to gauge with confidence the linguistic deficit in these officer-patients because he know how they *should* be able to speak, read, and write . . . they were the sort of men with whom he had mixed all his adult life; they were, in short, *gentlemen*. This ascription of status had important consequences for the form and content of Head's case histories . . . . Non-commissioned patients, on the other hand, were denied this unquestioned capacity to separate what was normal from what was pathological in their minds." L. S. Jacyna, *Medicine and Modernism: A Biography of Sir Henry Head* (London: Pickering and Chatto, 2008), 155.

10 Head, *Aphasia and Kindred Disorders of Speech*, I.147.

11 Jacyna, *Lost Words*, 153.

12 Jacyna, *Lost Words*, 150. See also Jacyna, *Medicine and Modernism*. This literary side is not entirely surprising, considering the fact that Head was himself a published poet and had assisted his wife Ruth in the editing of a collection of Thomas Hardy's poetry. See chapter on Henry Head in Rose, F. Clifford, ed., *Neurology of the Arts: Painting Music Literature* (London: Imperial College Press, 2004).

13 Peter Leese, *Shell Shock: Traumatic Neurosis and the British Soldiers of the First World War* (Hampshire and New York: Palgrave Macmillan, 2002), 77.

14 Public Record Office: Mental Illness/Neurasthenia Casesheets, MH 106 2102, Medical Case Notes, Rifleman W. B., August 1916; Also cited in: Leese, *Shell Shock*, 96.

15 Leese, *Shell Shock*, 36.

16 In 1916, Peter Leese notes, the Medical correspondent of the *Times* declared shell shock not a true disease but rather a "failure of willpower and loss of self-control." Leese, *Shell Shock*, 60.

17 Leese, *Shell Shock*, 51–2.

18 "Gunner McPhail," in Leese, *Shell Shock*, 101. Originally published in *The Springfield War Hospital Gazette*, September 1916, 14.

19 Siegfried Sassoon, *Collected Poems 1908–1956* (London: Faber and Faber, 1984), 83.

20 While the neurogenic view would gradually give way to the psychogenic, it did persist throughout the War, due to the large number of cases, which stood "on the borderline of concussion and neurosis." Leese, *Shell Shock*, 78. As Peter Leese shows, others like Sir John Collie, in his role as a public advocate for shell-shocked soldiers, argued that while shell shock was best understood as a manifestation of neurasthenia, or nerve-exhaustion, it still "directly or indirectly, [was] the result of actual concussions." Leese, *Shell Shock*, 61.

21 Leese, *Shell Shock*, 78.

22 Ibid., 159.

23 S. Ferenczi, *Psycho-Analysis and the War Neuroses*, with introduction by Sigmund Freud (London; Vienna; New York: The International Psycho-Analytical Press, 1921), 6.

24 Ferenczi, *Psycho-Analysis and the War Neuroses*, 14.

25 Sigmund Freud, Introduction to *Psycho-Analysis and the War Neuroses*, by S. Ferenczi (London; Vienna; New York: The International Psycho-Analytical Press, 1921), 2.

26 "In the traumatic and war neuroses the ego of the individual protects itself from a danger that either threatens it from without, or is embodied in a form of the ego itself, in the transference neuroses of peace time the ego regards its own sexual hunger (libido) as a foe, the demands of which appear threatening to it. In both cases the ego fears an injury; in the one case through the sexual hunger (libido) and in the other from outside forces." Freud, Introduction to *Psycho-Analysis and the War Neuroses*, 3.

27 Ferenczi, *Psycho-Analysis and the War Neuroses*, 15.

28 In his discussion of viable treatment methods for the condition, Ferenczi reveals not only this recognizability of the shell shock victim but also the stigmatization they still faced, even among well-informed members of the public: "Out of this chaos of symptoms the "trembling" neurosis stands out through its frequency

and conspicuousness. You all know those pathetic creatures who hobble along through the streets with shaking knees, uncertain gait and peculiar motor disturbances. They give the impression of being helpless and incurable invalids; and yet experience shows that this traumatic form of illness is purely psychogenic. A single treatment with electricity and suggestion, a few hypnotic sittings are often sufficient in rendering these men capable of doing some work, if only temporarily and under certain conditions." Ferenczi, *Psycho-Analysis and the War Neuroses*, 14. Ferenczi's prognosis for the average shell shock victim turned out to be supremely overconfident. As with Head's aphasic soldiers, it often took years for the symptoms of shell shock to fully subside.

29 Paul Fussell, "Binary Vision," in *The Great War and Modern Memory* (Oxford and New York: Oxford University Press, 1977), 90–105.

30 Robert Graves, *Good-bye to All That* (New York: Anchor Books, 1998), 114.

31 Wilfred Owens, *The Collected Poems* (New York: A New Directions Book, Chatto and Windus Ltd., 1963), 55.

32 Graves, *Good-bye to All That*, 114.

33 Owens, *The Collected Poems*, 55.

34 Graves, *Good-bye to All That*, 249; 112.

35 Robert Graves, *Listener*, 15 July 1971, 74; Also cited in Fussell, *The Great War and Modern Memory*, 170. Because sleep is another act of self-preservation, Graves points out that he also learns to distinguish sounds he can afford to sleep through from those he cannot: "I found it easy now to sleep through bombardments; though vaguely conscious of the noise, I let it go by. Yet if anybody came to wake me for my watch, or shouted "Stand to!", I was always alert in a second." Graves, *Good-bye to All That*, 213.

36 Fussell, *The Great War and Modern Memory*, see Chapter 7.

37 John Milton, *Paradise Lost* (Harlow: Longman, an imprint of Pearson Education Limited, 1998), I.660–8, 100.

38 Milton, *Paradise Lost*, VI.208–12, 349.

39 Owens, *The Collected Poems*, 61–2.

40 Robert Graves, *Collected Poems* (London: Cassell Publishers Limited, 1975), 93.

41 Sassoon, *Collected Poems*, 75.

42 Ibid., 107.

43 Jon Silkin, ed., *The Penguin Book of First World War Poetry* (London: Penguin Books, 1996), 116.

44 Silkin, *The Penguin Book of First World War Poetry*, 102.

45 Ibid., 116.

46 Sassoon, *Collected Poems*, 13.

47 Owens, *The Collected Poems*, 59.

48 Ibid., 44.

49 This ironic approach to the theme of noise offers yet another important example of what Paul Fussell identifies in *The Great War and Modern Memory* as the War poets' tendency toward dichotomizing, what he calls "a persisting imaginative habit of modern times, traceable, it would seem, to the actualities of the Great War," in which virtually everything is understood in terms of polar opposites and antitheses: "Us versus them," "Over here versus back there," etc. Fussell, *The Great War and Modern Memory*, 75. We have already seen how Graves and others formulated their experience of noise in ambivalent terms, as both threatening and life-preserving. It is David Jones, however, in his memoir *In Parenthesis*, who best expresses how noise was always understood in relation to its opposite: "I think the day by day in the Waste Land, the sudden violences and long stillnesses, the sharp contours and unformed voids of that mysterious existence, profoundly affected the imaginations of those who suffered it." Jones goes on to quote another war writer, Sir Thomas Malory, whose Arthurian battlegrounds are said to speak "with a grimly voice," to describe the common experience of long periods of silence suddenly interrupted by violent cacophonies. David Jones, *In Parenthesis* (New York: Penguin Books, 1963), 202. Also cited in Fussell, *The Great War and Modern Memory*, 144.

50 Silkin, *The Penguin Book of First World War Poetry*, 89–90; Sassoon, *Collected Poems*, 78.

51 Leese, *Shell Shock*, 61.

52 Wilfred Owens, *Collected Letters*, ed. Harold Owen and John Bell (London: Oxford University Press, 1967), 453.

53 Owens, *Collected Letters*, 456.

54 Daniel Hipp, *The Poetry of Shell Shock: Wartime Trauma and Healing in Wilfred Owen, Ivor Gurney and Siegfried Sassoon* (Jefferson, North Carolina and London: McFarland & Company, Inc., 2005), 57.

55 See Meredith Martin, "Therapeutic Measures: The Hydra and Wilfred Owen at Craiglockhart War Hospital." *Modernism*/Modernity 14, 1 (Jan 2007): 35–54; and Hipp, *The Poetry of Shell Shock*.

56 Wilfred Owens, "Editorial," in *Hydra*, 1 September (Edinborough: H. & J. Pillans & Wilson, Printers, 1917), 1.

57 Owens, "Editorial," in *Hydra*, 1.

58 Hipp, *The Poetry of Shell Shock*, 59–60.

59 Ibid., 60.

60 Ibid., 56.

61 Owens, *The Collected Poems*, 41.

62 Ibid., 128.

63 Ibid., 67.

64 Ibid., 80.

65 Martin, "Therapeutic Measures," 48.

66 Owens, *The Collected Poems*, 80; see also Wordsworth and Coleridge, *Lyrical Ballads* (1798). (Oxford and New York: Oxford University Press, 1969), 23.

67 Owens, *The Collected Poems*, 80.

68 Wordsworth and Coleridge, *Lyrical Ballads*, 153; 169.

69 Owens, *Collected Letters*, 431.

70 Ibid., 493.

71 Ibid., 60.

72 Ibid., 59.

73 ". . . he recalls and imagines beauty in the curses because of their function in uniting the men as expressions of communal courage." Hipp, *The Poetry of Shell Shock*, 86; See "Apologia Pro Poemate Meo," in Owens, *The Collected Poems*, 39.

74 Owens, *The Collected Poems*, 61; 74; 104; 85; 128.

75 Ibid., 85.

76 Ibid., 44.

77 Ibid., 128.

78 Ibid., 61.

79 Ibid., 427–8.

80 Hipp, *The Poetry of Shell Shock*, 48.

81 Owens, *The Collected Poems*, 61.

82 Graves, *Good-bye to All That*, 112.

83 Owens, *The Collected Poems*, 61.

84 Hipp, *The Poetry of Shell Shock*, 52.

85 Sassoon, *Collected Poems*, 19.

Chapter 3

1 Geoffrey O'Hara, "K-K-K-Katy: The Sensational Stammering Song Success Sung by Soldiers and Sailors," Performed by Billy Murray, Edison Records, 1917. (Check referencing)

2   See Gilbert Frankenau's *Peter Jackson, Cigar Merchant* (1920), A. P. Herbert's
    The Secret Battle (1919), Dorothy L. Sayers' *Whose Body?* (1923) and *Busman's
    Honeymoon* (1937), and Rebecca West's *The Return of the Soldier* (1918); Also
    cited in Leese, *Shell Shock*, 164–5.

3   *The Report of the War Office Committee of Enquiry into "Shell Shock,"* in the
    Wellcome Library for the History and Understanding of Medicine, RAMC
    Historical Collection, Ref. RAMC/739/19; Also cited in Leese, *Shell Shock*,
    166.

4   Virginia Woolf, *Mrs. Dalloway* (San Diego; New York; London: A Harvest Book,
    Harcourt Inc., 1981), 91–2.

5   Woolf, *Mrs. Dalloway*, 96.

6   Ibid., 183.

7   Ibid., 88.

8   Ibid., 98.

9   Ibid., 84.

10 Ibid., 84–5.

11 Ibid., 84.

12 Bobrick even claims that Freud was even "unwilling to treat stutterers since (in
    his view) psychoanalysis had failed to cast light on the disorder," but this is not
    exactly correct. Benson Bobrick, *Knotted Tongues: Stuttering in History and the
    Quest for a Cure* (New York: Kodansha International, 1995), 122. Whether it is
    accurate or not that Freud made it a general policy not to treat stuttering *per
    se* in the role of a psychoanalytic speech therapist, one of Freud's better-known
    hysterical patients did in fact speak with a stammer, and he did spend several
    weeks treating her stammer as one of her many hysterical symptoms. In 1889,
    Freud treated Frau Emmy Von M. for hysterical symptoms which included
    speech disturbances: "She spoke in a low voice as though with difficulty and
    her speech was from time to time subject to spastic interruptions amounting
    to a stammer." Joseph Breur and Sigmund Freud, *Studies on Hysteria*, trans.
    James Strachey (New York: Basic Books, 2000), 48–9.

13 Sandor Ferenczi, *Thalassa: A Theory of Genitality* (New York: Norton &
    Company, 1968), 7.

14 Ferenczi, *Thalassa*, 7.

15 Ibid., 9.

16 Ibid., 8–9.

17 Freud in Bobrick, *Knotted Tongues*, 122.

18 Isador H. Coriat, "The Psychoanalytic Conception of Stammering." *The Nervous Child* 2, 2 (1943): 167–71. See chapter 6 of Bobrick's *Knotted Tongues* for a more comprehensive history of psychoanalytic approaches to stuttering.

19 I. Peter Glauber, "Psychoanalytic Concepts of the Stutter." *The Nervous Child* 2, 2 (1943): 180.

20 Coriat, "The Psychoanalytic Conception of Stammering," 170.

21 Coriat, "The Psychoanalytic Conception of Stammering," 168; See also Robert West and Merle Ansberry, *The Rehabilitation of Speech* (New York: Harper and Row, 1968), 129.

22 Bobrick, *Knotted Tongues*, 121.

23 Robert Faggen, Introduction to *One Flew over the Cuckoo's Nest*, by Ken Kesey (New York: Penguin Books, 2002), xxii.

24 Herman Melville, *Billy Budd Sailor (An Inside Narrative)*, ed. Harrison Hayford and Merton M. Sealts Jr. (Chicago: University of Chicago Press, 1962), 50.

25 Melville, *Billy Budd*, 51; 52.

26 David Greven, "Flesh in the Word: *Billy Budd, Sailor,* Compulsory Homosociality, and the Uses of Queer Desire." *Genders* 37 (2003): 40.

27 Eve Kosofsky Sedgwick, *Epistemology of the Closet* (Berkeley: University of California Press, 2008), 103.

28 Melville, *Billy Budd*, 82.

29 Ibid.

30 Ibid., 98.

31 Richard Chase, "Innocence and Infamy," in *Herman Melville: A Critical Study* (New York: Macmillan, 1949), 258–77; Charles Olson, *Call Me Ishmael* (New York: Reynal and Hitchcock, 1947); Samuel Otter, "Introduction: Melville and Disability." *Leviathan* 8, 1 (2006): 7–16.

32 Melville, *Billy Budd*, 82; 53.

33 *The Oxford English Dictionary*, prepared by J. A. Simpson and E. S. C. Weiner (Oxford: Clarendon Press; New York: Oxford University Press, 1989).

34 Melville, *Billy Budd*, 68; 131.

35 Ibid., 71; 79.

36 Ibid., 84; 90.

37 Ibid., 74; 90.

38 Ibid., 56.

39 Melville, *Billy Budd*, 77; 72; John Wenke, "Melville's Indirection: *Billy Budd,* the Genetic Text, and the Deadly Space Between," in *New Essays on Billy Budd*, ed. Donald Yanella (Cambridge: Cambridge University Press, 2002), 126.

40 Melville, *Billy Budd*, 49.

41 Ibid., 92.

42 Ibid.

43 Ibid., 72.

44 Ibid., 79; 99.

45 Ibid., 99.

46 *The Oxford English Dictionary*.

47 Melville, *Billy Budd*, 47.

48 Ibid., 106.

49 Ken Kesey, *One Flew Over the Cuckoo's Nest* (New York: Penguin Books, 2002), 115.

50 Kesey, *Cuckoo's Nest*, 115.

51 Ibid., 272.

52 Ibid., 43.

53 Ibid., 194.

54 Ibid., 44; 93; 57.

55 Ibid., 5.

56 Ibid., 182.

57 Ibid.

58 Ibid., 117.

59 Noam Chomsky, *Syntactic Structures* (Berlin: Walter de Gruyter, 2002), 15.

60 Kesey, *Cuckoo's Nest*, 253.

61 Ibid.

62 Sigmund Freud, "Three Essays on the Theory of Sexuality," in *The Freud Reader*, ed. Peter Gay (New York: Norton, 1989), 292.

63 Kesey, *Cuckoo's Nest*, 254.

64 Ibid., 89.

65 Ibid., 118.

66 "Oh Helen," performed by Arthur Fields and Chorus (Edison Records, 1919).

67 Cliff Friend and Billy Rose, "You Tell her I Stutter," performed by the Happiness Boys (1923).

68 Marc Shell, *Stutter* (Cambridge, MA: Harvard University Press, 2005), 144; "Goody Groaner: The Celebrated Stammering Glee" (Eighteenth century ballad).

69 Shell, *Stutter*, 22.

70 J. L. Austin, *How To Do Things With Words*, 2nd edn, William James Lectures (New York; London: Oxford University Press, 1975).

71 Kesey, *Cuckoo's Nest*, 116.

72 Ibid., 81; 11.

73 Ibid., 187.

74 Ibid., 256.

75 Ibid., 270–1.

76 Ibid., 115.

77 Ibid., 265.

78 See the entry on momism in *American Masculinities: A Historical Encyclopedia*, ed. Bret Carroll (New York: SAGE, 2003), 318.

79 Philip Wylie, *Generation of Vipers* (New York: Dalkey Archive Press, 2007), 208.

80 Wylie, *Generation of Vipers*, 201.

81 Kesey, *Cuckoo's Nest*, 60; 64.

82 Wylie, *Generation of Vipers*, 216; Kesey, *Cuckoo's Nest*, 54.

83 Yukio Mishima, *Kinkaku-ji* (Tokyo: Shinchōsha, 1974), 7 (Japanese); Yukio Mishima, *The Temple of the Golden Pavilion,* trans. Ivan Morris (New York: Vintage, 1994), 7 (English).

84 Mishima, *The Temple of the Golden Pavilion*, 7.

85 Ibid., 5.

86 David Pollack, "Action as Fitting Match to Knowledge: Language and Symbol in Mishima's *Kinkakuji." Monumenta Nipponica* 40, 4, (1985): 395.

87 Mishima, *The Temple of the Golden Pavilion*, 40.

88 Rio Otomo, "'A Manifestation of Modernity: The Split Gaze and the Oedipalised Space of *The Temple of the Golden Pavilion* by Mishima Yukio." *Japanese Studies* 23, 3 (2003).

89 Otomo, "A Manifestation of Modernity," 277.

90 Mishima, *The Temple of the Golden Pavilion* (New York: Vintage, 1994).

91 Mishima, *The Temple of the Golden Pavilion*, 60.

92 Ibid., 88.

93 Ibid., 227–8.

94 Ibid., 12.

95 Yukio Mishima, *Sun and Steel*, trans. John Bester (New York: Kodansha, 1980), 10.

96 Mishima, *Sun and Steel*, 65.

97 Mishima, *The Temple of the Golden Pavilion*, 9.

98 Ibid., 142.

99 Ibid., 217.

100 Ibid., 247–8.

101 Graham Greene's 1958 novel *Our Man in Havana* offers yet another amalgamation of the many stereotypes of the Stutterer we've seen so far— neurotic, sexually timid, yet capable of violence—in the minor character of William Carter. *Our Man in Havana* is the story of James Wormold, a vacuum cleaner salesman who agrees to work for the British spy agency MI6. Although Wormold only submits falsified reports to London, his presence in Havana still attracts attention, eventually making Wormold a target for the assassin Carter. After gaining Wormold's trust, Carter poisons a glass of whisky and then offers it to Wormold. The sudden trace of a guilty stutter in Carter's speech makes Wormold suspicious: "'H-hurry,' Carter said. "You've got to h-hurry." Wormold lowered the whisky. "What did you say, Carter?"" Graham Greene, *Our Man in Havana* (London: Vintage Books, 2006), 180. Already aware that men are after him, Wormold pretends to accidentally tip the drink over. He then plots to kill Carter before Carter kills him. One night, Wormold invites the stuttering assassin to accompany him to a brothel. On the way, he finds out that Carter is "shy with women" Greene, *Our Man in Havana*, 206. When they reach the entrance to the brothel, Carter's confidence leaves him entirely: "With his hand on the door Carter paused again. He said, 'Perhaps it would be more sensible – some other night. You know, I h-h-h-h . . .' 'You are frightened, Carter.' 'I've never been to a h-h-h-house before. To tell you the truth, Wormold, I don't h-have much need with women'" Greene, *Our Man in Havana*, 207.

Chapter 4

1 One of the quintessential stagings of the people's voice as the voice that stutters comes in Robert Penn Warren's satire of American politics, *All The King's Men* (1946). Set in the Deep South in the 1930s, the novel follows the ascent of Willie Stark, whose right-hand man Sugar-Boy epitomizes the stereotype we outlined at the end of the previous chapter of the twitchy, violent stutterer. The awe that Sugar-Boy feels for Willie Stark stems predictably from Willie's gift for public speaking, and the impact of Willie's eloquence on an audience is described by Sugar-Boy in fittingly destructive terms: "'He could t-t-talk so good,' Sugar-Boy half-mumbled with his stuttering. 'The B-B-Boss could. Couldn't nobody t-t-talk like him. When he m-m-made a speech and ev-ev-everybody y-y-yelled, it looked l-l-like something was gonna b-b-burst inside y-y-you'"

Warren, *All the King's Men* (New York: Harcourt Books, 1974), 635. Through his speech impediment, Sugar-Boy can be said to stand for what Warren calls at one point "the tongue-tied population of honest men," that is, the populace who (like Owen's reticent soldiers) lack the ability or the desire to speak for themselves and for whom the eloquent politician must step in as their elected voice. Warren, *All the King's Men*, 95. After Willie is assassinated while giving a speech at the State Capitol, the narrator Jack Burden asks Sugar-Boy what he would do to the people behind the murder, to which Sugar-Boy replies without a single trace of a stutter, "I'd kill the son-of-a-bitch," again reflecting the notion one finds in virtually every stuttering narrative (from *Billy Budd* to *American Pastoral*) that physical violence in some way alleviates the stutter. Warren, *All the King's Men*, 633.

2 James Joyce, *Critical Writings*, ed. Ellsworth Mason and Richard Ellmann (New York: Cornell University Press, 1989), 225.

3 Robert Graves, *I, Claudius* (New York: Vintage International, 1989), 7.

4 Graves, *I, Claudius*, 52.

5 Ibid., 53.

6 Ibid., 52.

7 Ibid., 55.

8 Ibid., 14.

9 Ibid., 54.

10 Graves, *I, Claudius*, 55.

11 Ibid.

12 Graves, *I, Claudius*, 100.

13 Ibid., 62.

14 Ibid., 67.

15 Ibid., 125.

16 Robert Graves, *Claudius the God and his wife Messalina* (New York: Vintage International, 1989), 180. Xenophon treats him nonetheless, diagnosing his whole pathology as "a typical bryony case," and the regimen that eventually cures him, "bryony, massage, diet," again comically undercuts his lifelong disabilities: "Well, bryony cured me. For the first time in my life I knew what it was to be perfectly well. I followed Xenophon's advice to the letter and have hardly had a day's illness since. Of course, I remain lame and occasionally I stammer and twitch my head from old habit if I get excited. But my aphasia has disappeared, my hand hardly trembles at all." Graves, *Claudius the God and his wife Messalina*, 184.

17 Graves, *I, Claudius*, 69.

18 Ibid., 3.

19 Ibid., 9.

20 Ibid., 30.

21 Ibid., 210.

22 Ibid., 8.

23 Ibid., 7.

24 Ibid., 68.

25 Jean-Paul Forster, "The Gravesian Poem or Language Ill-Treated." *English Studies: A Journal of English Language and Literature* 60 (1979). In this article Forster elucidates the "analytical character" of Robert Graves' poetry, and its similarity to ordinary language philosophy, in particular, the twentieth-century analytic philosophers like Russell, Austin, and Wittgenstein. As Forster explains, for many of these analytic philosophers of language, "The business of philosophy came to be viewed as one of clarification rather than discovery, and its subject-matter increasingly our thought or language rather than the facts they expressed. In the case of Graves, the same assumption led the poet to consider his poems as attempts at clarifications rather than moments of discoveries, or even explorations." Forster, "The Gravesian Poem or Language Ill-Treated," 472. As examples of this clarifying approach to poetry, Forster cites poems like "Nature's Lineaments," "In Broken Images," and naturally "The Cool Web." What these poems have in common, for Forster, is a Wittgensteinean sense of the treacherousness of language, as well as an Austinian sense that the goal of poetry should be the demystification and disambiguation of language generally. In this respect, Forster writes, in Graves's poems, the investigation and clarification of facts is at the same time an investigation of language itself." Forster, "The Gravesian Poem or Language Ill-Treated," 473. Needless to say, this poetics of clarity and simplicity set him apart from most of his contemporaries, and the importance placed on clear language is something that carried over from his poetry to his prose writings on Claudius.

26 Graves, *I, Claudius*, 232.

27 Graves, *Claudius the God and his Wife Messalina*, 427.

28 Graves, *I, Claudius*, 466.

29 Ibid.

30 Graves, *Claudius the God and his Wife Messalina*, 344.

31 Ibid., 348.

32 Ibid., 432.

33   Ibid., 215–16.

34   In *Speech and Speech Disorders in Western Thought Before 1600*, Ynez
Viole O'Neill describes the legal implications of conditions like mutism
and stammering for Roman society. "Speechlessness," writes O'Neill, "was
considered to be a legal impediment, and speech was held to be a condition
requisite for full Roman citizenship." O'neill, *Speech and Speech Disorders in
Western Thought Before 1600* (London: Greenwood Press, 1980), 84. As O'Neill
shows, this gave mutes in Roman society the same legal status as children who,
as *infans*, were considered legally incapable because they were not yet in full
possession of their ability to speak and reason. Moreover, under the Justinian
Code, deaf-mutes were not allowed to give testimony and were excluded from
making oral contracts and other spoken transactions.

35   Ehud Yairi, Nicoline Ambrose and Nancy Cox, "Genetics of Stuttering: A
Critical Review." *Journal of Speech and Hearing Research* 39 (1996): 771–84.

36   Philip Roth, *American Pastoral* (New York: Vintage Press, 1998), 68.

37   Roth, *American Pastoral*, 243.

38   Ibid., 226.

39   Ibid., 95–6.

40   Coriat, "The Psychoanalytic Conception of Stammering," 170.

41   Roth, *American Pastoral*, 96.

42   Ibid., 97.

43   Ibid., 96.

44   Ibid., 90.

45   Ibid., 86.

46   Ibid., 86; 279.

47   Ibid., 91; 89.

48   Ibid., 91.

49   Ibid., 100; 103.

50   Ibid., 101.

51   Glauber, "Psychoanalytic Concepts of the Stutter," 178.

52   Roth, *American Pastoral*, 97.

53   Ibid., 101.

54   Ibid., 107.

55   Ibid., 106.

56   Ibid., 109.

57   Ibid., 240.

58 Ibid., 206.

59 Ibid., 100.

60 Ibid., 214.

61 West and Ansberry, *The Rehabilitation of Speech*, 128.

62 Roth, *American Pastoral*, 98.

63 Ibid., 99.

64 Edward Alexander, "Philip Roth at Century's End." *New England Review* 20, 2 (1999): 184. For more on the relationship between *American Pastoral* and 1960s political battles, see also Parrish and McCann. As McCann writes: "If the great stories of presidential imagination had imagined violence and coercion redeemed by the achievement of a renewed national compact, Roth's late fiction denies the promise of that resolution. Indeed, it suggests that the very pursuit of the pastoral dream of democratic community demands the coercion and repression, and produces the resentment, that will ultimately destroy it." Sean McCann, *A Pinnacle of Feeling: American Literature and Presidential Government* (Princeton, NJ: Princeton University Press, 2008), 191.

65 Sandra Kumamoto Stanley, "Mourning the 'Greatest Generation': Myth and History in Philip Roth's *American Pastoral.*" *Twentieth Century Literature* 51, 1 (2005): 3.

66 Stanley, "Myth and History in Philip Roth's *American Pastoral,*" 6.

67 Roth, *American Pastoral*, 279. Another precursor to Merry's rapid-fire stuttering is the character of Wendell Kretschmar in Thomas Mann's *Doktor Faustus* (1947). Kretschmar is a German-American music scholar from Pennsylvania who lectures to the novel's protagonist Adrian Leverkuhn in a severe stutter about Bach and other musical subjects. During his lectures, Kretschmar's stutter reaches a severity that Mann likens to machine-gun fire: "Kretschmar began to stutter violently, holding on to its initial consonant, his tongue set up a kind of machine-gun fire against his palate, setting jaw and chin pulsing in sync, before they came to rest in the vowel that allowed one to surmise the rest." Mann, *Doctor Faustus: The Life of the German Composer Adrian Leverkühn As Told by a Friend* (New York: Vintage International, 1999), 57.

68 Roth, *American Pastoral*, 73.

69 Ibid., 259.

70 Ibid., 86.

71 Gail Jones, *Sorry* (London: Harvill Secker, 2007), 8.

72 Gail Jones, *Sorry*, 4.

73 Ibid., 63.

74 Ibid., 32.

75 Ibid., 103.

76 Ibid., 151.

77 Ibid., 213.

78 Ibid., 96.

79 Ibid., 182.

80 Ibid., 100.

81 Ibid., 212.

82 Ibid., 166.

83 Ibid., 31.

84 Ibid., 109.

85 Ibid., 151; 31.

86 Ibid., 156.

87 Ibid., 182.

88 Ibid., 141.

89 Ibid., 175.

90 Ibid., 173.

91 Ibid., 193.

92 Ibid., 195.

93 Ibid., 56.

94 Ibid., 205.

95 In 2007, Kevin Rudd did offer a formal apology as his first act as Prime Minister.

96 Gail Jones, "Sorry-in-the-Sky: Empathetic Unsettlement, Mourning, and the Stolen Generations," in *Imagining: Literature and Culture in the New New World*, ed. Judith Ryan and Chris Wallace-Crabbe (Cambridge, MA: Harvard University Press, 2004), 164.

97 Gail Jones, "Sorry-in-the-Sky: Empathetic Unsettlement, Mourning, and the Stolen Generations," 165.

98 Ibid.

99 Ibid.

100 Gail Jones, *Sorry*, 204.

101 For a fascinating example of forensic profiling of the Stutterer, see John Douglas's book *Mind Hunter: Inside the FBI's Serial Crime Unit*. In the chapter entitled "The Killer Will Have A Speech Impediment," Douglas describes his involvement in the manhunt of the Trailside Killer, the serial killer David

Carpenter who murdered women on hiking trails near San Francisco. As part of his profile, Douglas correctly predicted that the Trailside Killer would be someone who spoke with a severe stutter. Douglas, *Mind Hunter: Inside the FBI's Serial Crime Unit* (New York: Pocket Books, 2003).

102 Political activism and the building of bombs only provide a temporary cure for Merry's stutter, and it is not until she converts to Jainism that the final traces of her speech disorder are removed. Replacing the destructive act of building bombs, Merry's strict adherence to the moral codes of Jainism stands as a form of nonviolent protest. In striving to achieve a "perfected soul . . . through the rigors of asceticism and self-denial and through the doctrine of *ahimsa* or nonviolence," Merry continues to reject her father's perfectionist demands, but her chosen mode of expression now entails relinquishing identity altogether. Her former rage which manifested externally as bombs is now directed toward the violent destruction of her own body, and "everything angry inside her had broken into the open." Gail Jones, *Sorry*, 232; 249.

Chapter 5

1 Jean M. G. Itard, "Mémoire sur Quelques Fonctions Involontaires des Appareils de la Locomotion, de la Préhension et de la Voix." *Archives Générales de Médecine* 8 (1825): 405.

2 Georges Gilles de la Tourette, "Etude sur une Affection Nerveuse Caracterisee par de l'Incoordination Motrice Accompagnee d'Echolalie et de Coprolalie." *Archives de Neurologie* 9 (1885): 26; 180.

3 Ernest Billod, "Maladies de la Volonté." (three part study), *Annales Médico-Psychologiques* 10, 1 (1847); Also cited in Howard I. Kushner, *A Cursing Brain* (Boston: Harvard University Press, 2000), 7.

4 Théodule Ribot, *Les Maladies de la Volonté*, 14th ed. (Paris: Félix Alcan, 1883), 55.

5 Kushner, *A Cursing Brain*, 26.

6 For Brissaud, ticcishness was "no more than than the superlative expression of a neuropathic and psychopathic disposition." Professor Édouard Brissaud, preface to *Tics and their Treatment*, by Henry Meige and E. Feindel (New York: William Wood and Company, 1907); Also cited in Kushner, *A Cursing Brain*, 48.

7 Kushner, *A Cursing Brain*, 48.

8   In *A Cursing Brain*, Kushner notes that Ferenczi was not the very first to put forward this theory that tics were related to masturbatory urges. To be precise, Kushner points out earlier work by J. C. Wilson and Otto Lerch who "had connected masturbation with tics and coprolalia, *but* they had argued that ticcers were *actual* masturbators." Kushner, *A Cursing Brain*, 62.

9   Kushner, *A Cursing Brain*, 62. Kushner points out the obvious paradox that this creates from a psychoanalytic viewpoint, since the standard Freudian account of catatonia, the polar opposite of ticcishness, was that it also stemmed from sexual repression: "If, as Ferenczi insisted, all tics had the same root, a reaction against a repressed libido, how were tics to be distinguished from their seeming opposite manifestation of catatonia, a rigidity and lack of movement which had been explained by Freud as also resulting from dammed-up libido? The answer, in classic psychoanalytic style, was that these were two opposite outcomes resulting from the same underlying causes." Kushner, *A Cursing Brain*, 63.

10   Oliver Sacks, *The Man Who Mistook His Wife for a Hat and Other Clinical Tales* (New York: Touchstone, 1998), 3.

11   Sacks, *The Man Who Mistook His Wife for a Hat*, 87.

12   Jonathan Lethem, *Motherless Brooklyn* (New York: First Vintage Contemporaries, 2000), 204.

13   Lethem, *Motherless Brooklyn*, 46.

14   Ibid., 48.

15   Ronald Schleifer, "The Poetics of Tourette Syndrome: Language, Neurobiology, and Poetry." *New Literary History* 32, 3 (Summer 2001): 574; See Ruth D. Bruun, "The Natural History of Tourette's Syndrome," in *Tourette's Syndrome and Tic Disorders*, eds. Donald J. Cohen, Ruth D. Bruun, James F. Leckman (New Jersey: Wiley-Interscience, 1988), 21–39, esp. 22–5.

16   Lethem, *Motherless Brooklyn*, 42.

17   Ibid., 45.

18   Ibid., 47.

19   Ibid., 81.

20   Ibid., 82.

21   Oliver Sacks, *An Anthropologist on Mars* (New York: Vintage, 1996), 81.

22   Lethem, *Motherless Brooklyn*, 82.

23   Ibid., 258; 220.

24   Ibid., 118.

25 This mental compartmentalization is what allows Lionel to make the remark during his stakeout of the L&L that "a sentinel part of my brain had kept watch while the rest of me slept." Lethem, *Motherless Brooklyn*, 249. This remark is just one of many examples showing how the multiple tracks working at once inside Lionel's brain are described in neurological terms. In addition to this segregation of brain and self, Lionel's brain is sometimes further fragmented within itself, such that when Lionel is being questioned by four thugs, he is able to note that, "one part of my brain was thinking, *Handle with scare, scandal with hair*, and so on. Another part was puzzling over the Tony question." Lethem, *Motherless Brooklyn*, 151. What these examples are intended to suggest is an entirely different understanding of the neural self.

26 Another relevant example of this comes during one of his conversations with Kimmery. Lionel struggles to control his physical compulsion to adjust Kimmery's collar, while "My brain went, *How are you feeling and how are you thinking and think how you're feeling*." Lethem, *Motherless Brooklyn*, 217. In this scene, not only does Lionel's tourettic brain exercise its own agency of speech, but it is also able to address Lionel directly and, as it were, personally. The sense of powerlessness that comes from this even leads Lionel at one point to "beg [his] Tourette's self" not to exhibit a verbal or physical tic. Lethem, *Motherless Brooklyn*, 22.

27 The novel's two protagonists, Thérèse and Laurent, are presented in strictly deterministic terms as biological organisms without soul or free will, governed entirely by their heredity and environment. Thérèse's inherently nervous temperament is inevitably drawn to Laurent's inherently sanguine temperament, and the couple's absence of willpower is confirmed through Zola's portrayal of their status as a single unified organism. For instance, in the planning of Camille's murder, Thérèse and Laurent are reduced to a single brain: "They dared not peer down to the depths of their being, to the depths of this feverish confusion which filled their brain with a sort of dense, acrid mist [Eux-mêmes n'osaient regarder au fond de leur être, au fond de cette fièvre trouble qui emplissait leur cerveau d'une sorte de vapeur épaisse et âcre]." Zola, *Thérèse Raquin* (London: Penguin Books, 1962), 86 (my translation). In addition to the singularizing of their shared brain (leur cerveau, rather than leurs cerveaux), it is significant that Zola does not refer to the couple's bond in their plan to murder Camille as a shared "esprit," which would suggest a higher (psychological or spiritual) sense of mind or spirit. Instead, he chooses the more

strictly anatomical term "cerveau" to indicate that their mental state, as well as their decision-making, is merely the product of a shared neurophysiology. Their murder of Camille is thus described deterministically as the necessary and inevitable culmination of their animalistic urges.

28 Lethem, *Motherless Brooklyn*, 2.

29 Zola, *Thérèse Raquin*, trans. Andrew Rothwell (Oxford: Oxford University Press World's Classics, 1992), 153.

30 Zola, *Thérèse Raquin* (Oxford: Oxford University Press World's Classics, 1992), 153.

31 Ibid.

32 The emphasis in this passage on Laurent's inability to control his own hand is again framed in terms of willpower, or lack thereof. It is not imagination, talent, or painterly skill that allows Laurent to produce these strange masterpieces. Rather, it is the introduction of Thérèse's nerves into his sanguine body that makes it possible, and Laurent's artistic activity is performed compulsively, not freely. Laurent is forced to conclude that he will never again be able to paint because "the thought that his fingers had an unavoidable and involuntary ability to keep on reproducing Camille's portrait made him stare at his hand in terror. It felt as if it no longer belonged to him." Zola, *Thérèse Raquin* (Oxford: Oxford University Press World's Classics, 1992), 154. Laurent's involuntary retracing of Camille's face culminates in the sensation that his hand is an autonomous entity separate from his own body.

33 Lethem, *Motherless Brooklyn*, 6.

34 Ibid., 20.

35 Ibid., 113.

36 Ibid., 112.

37 Ibid., 15.

38 Ibid., 131.

39 Ibid., 83.

40 Ibid., 131.

41 Lethem, *Motherless Brooklyn*, 15; 34; 174; 163; 42. In general, Lionel's "tics were always worst when [he] was nervous," and he can measure when his Tourette's is at its most severe when, for instance, he becomes "tic-gripped, helpless" during his phone conversation with the mobsters Matricardi and Rockaforte. Lethem, *Motherless Brooklyn*, 11; 64. In an earlier meeting with the same mobsters, Lionel is further able to determine the exact extent to which his motor activity

is in or out of his control when, in the middle of being questioned about Tony's whereabouts, he notes that, while he "wasn't exactly ticcing," he had begun to "echo The Clients' verbal rhythms." Lethem, *Motherless Brooklyn*, 174. When in the company of Kimmery, Lionel feels "sheltered in her tic-canceling field" and is "conscious of his ticlessness" under her calming influence. Lethem, *Motherless Brooklyn*, 195; 136.

42 Lethem, *Motherless Brooklyn*, 211.
43 Ibid.
44 Lethem, *Motherless Brooklyn*, 11; 78.
45 Ibid., 299.
46 Ibid., 78.
47 Ibid., 216.
48 Ibid., 155.
49 Ibid., 57; 58.
50 Ibid., 171.
51 Ibid., 172.
52 Ibid., 47.
53 Ibid., 104.
54 Dorothy Hale, "As I Lay Dying's Heterogeneous Discourse." *NOVEL: A Forum on Fiction* 23, 1 (Autumn 1989): 5–23.
55 Lethem, *Motherless Brooklyn*, 8; 99; 116; 33; 155.
56 Ibid., 195.
57 Ibid., 82.
58 Ibid., 13.
59 Ibid., 27.
60 Ibid., 276.
61 Ibid., 259.
62 Ibid., 195.
63 Ibid., 109.
64 Ibid., 247.
65 Ibid., 263.
66 Ibid., 101.
67 Ibid., 149.
68 Ibid., 75.
69 Ibid., 114.
70 Ibid., 92.

71 Ibid., 34.

72 Ibid., 113.

73 A little later in the same scene, Lionel is interrogated by the homicide detective, who is tiring of Lionel's "double-talk." Lethem, *Motherless Brooklyn*, 115. Denying any knowledge of the mobsters Matricardi and Rockaforte, Lionel consciously exaggerates the severity of his syndrome, thinking to himself "let Tourette be the suspect and maybe I'd get off the hook." Lethem, *Motherless Brooklyn*, 110. When the detective doubts the truth behind Lionel's story, Lionel responds by saying, "Believemeblackman," a phrase that sounds like tourettic speech, but the lack of italics again implies that it is a free utterance. Lethem, *Motherless Brooklyn*, 115. Is Lionel engaging in wordplay here or deliberately trying to control situation by exploiting his own condition? The fact that Lionel is lying to the detective—both about his knowledge of the mobsters and about the acuteness of his tics—raises interesting questions concerning the relationship between language and lying. Lionel appears to be playing with his own verbal habits by imitating what one of his tics would probably sound like, but is his utterance a semicompulsive tic or an outright lie? Is he only partially in control of his speech or is he making a willed decision to hide the truth? The difficulty of determining the exact nature of this tic stems from the fact that, just as there are gradations between the various forms of Lionel's ticcishness, so too are there varying degrees of agency that Lionel is able to exert over his own speech.

74 Lethem, *Motherless Brooklyn*, 83.

75 Ibid., 47.

76 Ibid., 83.

77 Ibid., 57.

78 In my discussion in Chapter 3 on the interrelationship between stuttering and sexuality, I suggest that according to the psychogenic view of "organic hesitancy," the male stutterer often experiences temporary release from his blocked speech through the act of sexual ejaculation. Despite the cultural oppositions we have pointed out between stuttering and Tourette's, there is a similar connection made in *Motherless Brooklyn* between sexuality and Tourette's.

79 Lethem, *Motherless Brooklyn*, 103.

80 Ibid., 104.

81 Ibid., 182.

82 Ibid., 301.

83 Lethem, *Motherless Brooklyn*, 182. Another interesting scene in which sexuality is shown to temporarily cure Lionel's ticcishness occurs when Lionel goes with Kimmery to her apartment, following the commotion that takes place at the Zendo. In the "alleviating presence" of Kimmery, Lionel becomes sexually aroused and begins to mirror her gestures as she draws circles on his leg. Lethem, *Motherless Brooklyn*, 194. However, Lionel explicitly tells us that his act of mirroring is not an involuntary physical tic, but rather an intentional act: "I was never less ticcish than this: aroused, pressing toward another's body, moving out of my own. But just as Kimmery had somehow spared me ticcing aloud in conversation, I now felt free to incorporate an element of Tourette's into our groping, as though she were negotiating a new understanding between my two disgruntled brains." Lethem, *Motherless Brooklyn*, 220. Lionel's usual involuntary obsessive compulsive tapping is juxtaposed in this scene with his free touching of Kimmery's body. Through sexual pleasure, Lionel is thus able to exercise agency over his tourettic condition by voluntarily incorporating his tics into his touching. Interestingly, the only time in the novel when Lionel becomes opaque and "strange" to himself is this exact moment when his ticcishness disappears. Lethem, *Motherless Brooklyn*, 219. The hyperawareness he usually has regarding his tics is replaced by an absence of self-knowledge as he explores Kimmery's body: "Then her hand fell lower, and mine too, and at that moment I felt my hand and mind lose their particularity, their pointiness, their countingness, instead become clouds of general awareness." Lethem, *Motherless Brooklyn*, 220. Lionel becomes opaque to himself in this instant namely because the "particularity" of his Tourette's, with its polyphony of competing voices, gives way to a "generality," a single "stilled self" who is free of language: "I made a whining sound, not a part of any word. Language was destroyed." Lethem, *Motherless Brooklyn*, 222. Although Lionel reaches a state of wordlessness while having sex with Kimmery, his tics resurface soon after he orgasms: "From twitch to orgasm, the way sex first smoothed away tics, then supplanted them with a violent double: little death, big tic." Lethem, *Motherless Brooklyn*, 224. Lethem's reference here to the French euphemism "little death" (*la petite mort)* for orgasm confirms that, just as in the cases of Billy Bibbit and Mizoguchi, sexuality only offers a temporary cure for Lionel's Tourette's. His tics return in full force after his orgasm, and Lionel has come to expect "a punishment after sex." Lethem, *Motherless Brooklyn*, 224.

84 Lethem, *Motherless Brooklyn*, 137.

85 Ibid., 138.

86 Ibid., 214.

87 Ibid., 195.

88 Ibid.

89 Lethem, *Motherless Brooklyn*, 198. This farcical moment of Lionel becoming sexually stimulated in the middle of meditating perfectly highlights how impossible it would seem to be for a Tourette's sufferer to practice Zen sitting. Lionel's linking of his penis to the achievement of One Mind also brings us back to our earlier discussion of how sexual activity succeeds in stilling the multiple tracks in Lionel's mind, or as he puts it, "I'm still myself and still in myself." Lethem, *Motherless Brooklyn*, 198. This stilled state of being during sexual activity is the closest Lionel comes to achieving a Zen-like mental and physical stillness. Lionel even sees Kimmery as the unifying force between his "two disgruntled brains," suggesting that reaching orgasm is synonymous, for Lionel, with achieving One Mind. But ultimately, sex proves to be no more effective than *zazen* in producing any permanent cure for Lionel's Tourette's.

90 Lethem, *Motherless Brooklyn*, 160.

91 Ibid.

92 Ibid., 237.

93 Ibid., 264.

94 Ibid., 265.

95 Ibid., 264.

96 Oliver Sacks, "Tourette's syndrome and creativity: Exploiting the ticcy witticisms and witty ticcicisms." *BMJ* 305 (December 1992): 15.

97 Ronald Schleifer, "The Poetics of Tourette Syndrome: Language, Neurobiology, and Poetry." *New Literary History* 32, 3 (Summer 2001): 568.

98 Lethem, *Motherless Brooklyn*, 15.

99 Ibid., 2; 142; 33; 4.

100 Mikhail M. Bakhtin, *The Dialogic Imagination: Four Essays*, trans. Caryl Emerson and Michael Holquist (Austin: University of Texas Press, 1981), 311.

101 Bakhtin, *The Dialogic Imagination*, 293.

102 Ibid.

103 Ibid., 294.

104 Lethem, *Motherless Brooklyn*, 47.

105 Ibid., 309.

106 Bakhtin, *The Dialogic Imagination*, 324.

Conclusion

1 Jeffrey K. Johnson, "The Visualisation of the Twisted Tongue: Portrayals of Stuttering in Film, Television, and Comic Books." *The Journal of Popular Culture* 41, 2 (2008): 245.

2 Susan Sontag, *Illness as Metaphor and Aids and its Metaphors* (London: Penguin Modern Classics, 2002), 3.

3 Gilles Deleuze, "He Stuttered," in *Essays Critical and Clinical* (Minneapolis: University of Minnesota Press, 1997), 109.

4 Deleuze, "He Stuttered," 111.

5 Ibid., 107.

6 Ibid., 108.

7 Ibid.

8 Michel De Certeau, "Vocal Utopias: Glossolalias." *Representations* no.56, Special Issue: The New Erudition (Autumn 1996): 29.

9 De Certeau, "Vocal Utopias: Glossolalias," 32.

10 Ibid., 41.

11 Boris Eichenbaum, *Anna Akhmatova* cited in Victor Erlich, *Russian Formalism History – Doctrine* (Hague: Mouton & Co. Publishers, 1955), 256.

12 Victor Shklovksy, "Art as Technique," in *Russian Formalist Criticism: Four Essays*, eds. Lee T. Lemon and Marion J. Reis (London: University of Nebraska Press, 1965), 22.

13 No one is more culpable of this kind of reductionism than Jonah Lehrer, in his bestseller *Proust Was A Neuroscientist*. "We now know," Jonah Lehrer writes "that Proust was right about the memory." Lehrer, *Proust Was a Neuroscientist* (New York: Mariner Books, 2008), xi. Actually, we've known this for quite some time.

Bibliography

Adrian, E. D., and L. R. Yealland. "Treatment of War Neuroses." *The Lancet*, 9 June 1917, 867–72.

Albaret, Céleste. *Monsieur Proust.* Paris: Robert Laffont, 1973.

Alexander, Edward. "Philip Roth at Century's End." *New England Review* 20, 2 (1999): 183–90. http://search.proquest.com.

Austin, J. L. *How To Do Things With Words.* 2nd ed. William James Lectures. New York; London: Oxford University Press, 1975.

Bakhtin, Mikhail M. *The Dialogic Imagination: Four Essays.* Translated by Caryl Emerson and Michael Holquist. Austin: University of Texas Press, 1981.

Ball, Martin J. and Jack S. Damico. *Clinical Aphasiology: Future Directions.* Hove; New York: Psychology Press, Taylor & Francis Group, 2007.

Barker, Lewellys F. *The Nervous System and Its Constituent Neurones.* New York: Appleton, 1899.

—. *Time and the Physician: The Autobiography of Lewellys F. Barker.* New York: Putnam, 1942.

Barker, Pat. *Regeneration.* London: Penguin Books, 2009.

—. *The Ghost Road.* London: Penguin Books, 2010.

—. *The Eye in the Door.* London: Penguin Books, 1994.

Barthes, Roland. *Le degré zéro de l'écriture.* Paris: Éditions de Seuil, 1972a.

—. "Proust et les noms." *Le degré zéro de l'écriture suivi de Nouveaux essays critiques.* Paris: Éditions de Seuil, 1972b.

Bauby, Jean-Dominique. *The Diving Bell and the Butterfly.* New York: Vintage International, 1998.

Baudelaire, Charles. *Correspondance II (mars 1860-mars 1866).* Paris: Gallimard, 1973.

—. "L'aphasie." *Revue Neurologique* 125, 4 (1971): 310–6.

Bell, David F. "Thérèse Raquin: Scientific Realism in Zola's Laboratory." *Nineteenth Century French Studies* 24 (1995 Fall to 1996 Winter): 122–32. http://www.cat.inist.fr/?aModele=afficheN&cpsidt=3279611.

Benton, Arthur L. and Robert J. Joynt. "Early Descriptions of Aphasia." *Archives of Neurology* 3 (1960). Accessed 11 April 2010. http://www.archneurol.com.

Bergson, Henri. *Matter and Memory.* New York: Dover Publications Inc., 2004.

Bernard, Claude. *Introduction à l'étude de la médicine expérimentale.* Paris: Flammarion, 1952.

—. *An Introduction to the Study of Experimental Medicine.* New York: The Macmillan Company, 1927.

Bernard, Désiré. *De L'Aphasie et De Ses Diverses Formes.* Paris: Publications du Progrès Médical, Par Ch. Féré, Médicin de Bicêtre, 1889.

Beusterien, John. "Did Cervantes Stutter?" *Cervantes: Bulletin of the Cervantes Society of America* 29, 1 (2009): 209–20. http://www.dialnet.unirioja.es/servlet/articulo?codigo=3163380.

Billod, Ernest. "Maladies de la Volonté." (three part study) *Annales Médico-Psychologiques* 10, 1 (1847): 15–35; 170–202; 317–47.

Bobrick, Benson. *Knotted Tongues: Stuttering in History and the Quest for a Cure.* New York: Kodansha International, 1995.

Bogousslavsky, Julien, and Sebastian Dieguez. "Baudelaire's Aphasia: From Poetry to Cursing." In *Neurological Disorders in Famous Artists, Part 2,* edited by Julien Bogousslavsky and Frantois Boller. New York: Karger, 2007.

Bogousslavsky, Julien. *Following Charcot: A Forgotten History of Neurology and Psychiatry (Frontiers of Neurology and Neuroscience).* Zurich: S. Karger AG, 2011.

—. "Marcel Proust's Diseases and Doctors: The Neurological Story of a Life." In *Neurological Disorders in Famous Artists, Part 2,* edited by Julien Bogousslavsky and Frantois Boller. New York: Karger, 2007a, 89–104.

—. "Marcel Proust's Lifelong Tour of the Parisian Neurological Intelligentsia: From Brissaud and Dejerine to Sollier and Babinski." *European Neurology* 57 (January 2007b): 129–36. http://dx.doi.org.ezproxy.uws.edu.au/10.1159/000098463.

Bogue, Benjamin Nathaniel. *Stammering: Its Cause and Cure.* Chicago: Hammond Press, 1929.

Bonaddio, Federico. "Sensing the Stutter: A Stammerer's Perception of Lorca." *Neophilologus* 82 (1998): 53–62. doi:10.1023/A:1004285319904.

Boswell, James. *Life of Johnson: Unabridged.* Oxford: Oxford University Press, 1998.

Bouillaud, Jean-Baptiste. "Recherches Cliniques." *Archives Générales de Médicine* Paris 8 (1825): 25–45.

Breen, Jennifer. "Wilfred Owen (1893–1918): His Recovery from 'Shellshock.'" *Notes and Queries* 23 (July 1976): 301–5.

Breur, Joseph and Sigmund Freud. *Studies on Hysteria.* Translated by James Strachey. New York: Basic Books, 2000.

Brissaud, Professor Édouard. Preface to *Tics and their Treatment* by Henry Meige and E. Feindel. New York: William Wood and Company, 1907.

Broca, Paul. *Écrits sur l'aphashie (1861–1869): Introduction historique et textes réunis par Serge Nicolas.* Paris; Budapest; Torino: L'Harmattan, 2004.

Brookshire, Robert H. *Introduction to Neurogenic Communication Disorders.* New York: Mosby Press, 1997.

Brown, Jason W., ed., *Jargonaphasia.* New York: Academic Press, 1981.

Bruun, Ruth D. "The Natural History of Tourette's Syndrome." In *Tourette's Syndrome and Tic Disorders,* edited by Donald J. Cohen, Ruth D. Bruun and James F. Leckman. New Jersey: Wiley-Interscience, 1988, 21–39.

Buckingham, Hugh W. "Introductory essay: Perseveration happens!" *Aphasiology* 21 (2007): 916–27. doi:10.1080/02687030701198205.

—. "Was Sigmund Freud the first neogrammarian neurolinguist?" *Aphasiology* 20 (2006): 1085–1104. doi:10.1080/02687030600741626.

Buckingham, Hugh W. and Andrew Kertesz. *Neologistic Jargon Aphasia.* Amsterdam: Swets & Zeitlinger B. V., 1976.

Buss, Robin. Introduction to *Thérèse Raquin* by Émile Zola. London: Penguin Books, 2010.

Cantor, David. "Between Galen, Geddes, and the Gael: Arthur Brock, Modernity, and Medical Humanism in Early-Twentieth-Century Scotland." *Journal of the History of Medicine and Allied Sciences* 60, 1 (January 2005): 1–41. doi:10.1093/jhmas/jri001.

Caplan, David. *Neurolinguistics and Linguistic Aphasiology: An Introduction.* Cambridge: Cambridge University Press, 1987.

Carroll, Brett, ed., *American Masculinities: A Historical Encyclopedia.* New York: SAGE, 2003.

Carroll, Lewis. *Alice's Adventures in Wonderland* and *Through the Looking Glass.* New York: Penguin Books, 1998.

Carter, William C. *Marcel Proust: A Life.* New Haven; London: Yale University Press, 2000.

Changeux, Jean-Pierre. *Neuronal Man: The Biology of Mind.* Princeton, NJ: Princeton University Press, 1985.

Chase, Richard. "Innocence and Infamy." In *Herman Melville: A Critical Study.* New York: Macmillan, 1949, 258–77.

Chomsky, Noam. *Syntactic Structures.* Berlin: Walter de Gruyter, 2002.

Clarke, Bruce and Wendell Aycock, eds. *The Body and the Text: Comparative Essays in Literature and Medicine.* Lubbock, Texas: Texas Tech University Press, 1990.

Clifford, Rose, F., ed., *Neurology of the Arts: Painting Music Literature.* London: Imperial College Press, 2004.

Code, Chris, ed., *The Characteristics of Aphasia.* Philadelphia: Taylor and Francis, 1989.

Cohen, Henning. "The Singing Stammerer Motif in Billy Budd." *Western Folklore* 34, 1 (January 1975): 54–5. http://www.jstor.org.

Coriat, Isador H. "The Psychoanalytic Conception of Stammering." *The Nervous Child* 2, 2 (1943): 167–71. http://www.psycnet.apa.org.

Crépet, J. "Les derniers jours de Charles Baudelaire." *La Nouvelle Revue Française* 21 (1932): 641–71.

Critchley, Macdonald. "Dr. Samuel Johnson's Aphasia." *Medical History* 6, 1 (January 1962): 27–44. http://www.ncbi.nlm.nih.gov/pmc/. doi:PMC1034671.

Davis, Lennard J. *The Disability Studies Reader: Second Edition*. New York: Routledge, 2006.

De Certeau, Michel. "Vocal Utopias: Glossolalias." *Representations* no.56, Special Issue: The New Erudition (Autumn 1996): 29–47. doi:10.2307/2928706.

De La Tourette, Georges Gilles. "Etude sur une affection nerveuse caracterisee par de l'incoordination motrice accompagnee d'echolalie et de coprolalie." *Archives de Neurologie* 9 (1885): 19–42; 158–200.

De Man, Paul. *The Rhetoric of Romanticism*. New York: Columbia University Press, 1984.

Delamotte, Isabelle. "La place de Charcot dans la documentation médicale d'Émile Zola." *Cahiers Naturalistes* 73 (1999): 287–99. http://www.cat.inist.fr/?aModele=af ficheN&cpsidt=1553174.

Delaporte, Sophie. *Gueules Cassées de la Grande Guerre* [*The Shattered Faces of the Great War*]. Paris: Broché Épuisé, 2004.

Deleuze, Gilles. *Proust et les signes*. Paris: Presses Universitaire de Paris, 1998.

—. "He Stuttered." In *Essays Critical and Clinical*. Minneapolis: University of Minnesota Press, 1997.

Derrida, Jacques. "Des tours de Babel." *Difference in Translation*. Edited and translated by Joseph F. Graham. Ithaca: Cornell University Press, 1985.

Douglas, John. *Mind Hunter: Inside the FBI's Serial Crime* Unit. New York: Pocket Books, 2003.

Eagle, Christopher. "On 'This' and 'That' in Proust: Deixis and Typologies in *A la recherche du temps Perdu*." *MLN* 121 (2006): 989–108. http://www.jstor.org.

—. "Organic Hesitancies: Stuttering and Masculinity in Melville, Kesey, and Mishima." *Comparative Literature* 48, 2 (2011): 200–18. http://www. muse.jhu.edu/.

Eco, Umberto. *The Search for the Perfect Language*. Translated by James Fentress. Oxford: Blackwell Publishers, Inc., 1995.

Eggert, Gertrude H. *Wernicke's Works on Aphasia: A Sourcebook and Review: Early Sources in Aphasia and Related Disorders*. The Hague, Paris and New York: Mouton Publishers, 1977.

Eling, Paul, ed., *Reader in the History of Aphasia*. Philadelphia: John Benjamins Publishing Company, 1994.

Erlich, Victor. *Russian Formalism History – Doctrine*. Hague: Mouton & Co. Publishers, 1955.

Faggen, Robert. Introduction to *One Flew over the Cuckoo's Nest*, by Ken Kesey. New York: Penguin Books, 2002.

Farland, Marla. "Gertrude Stein's Brain Work." *American Literature* 76, 1 (March 2004): 117–48. http://www.muse.jhu.edu.

Ferenczi, S. *Psycho-Analysis and the War Neuroses*. With Introduction by Sigmund Freud. London; Vienna; New York: The International Psycho-Analytical Press, 1921, 1–21.

—. *Thalassa: A Theory of Genitality*. New York: Norton & Company, 1968.

Foucault, Michel. *Naissance de la Clinique*. Paris: Presses Universitaires de France, 2003.

—. *The Birth of the Clinic: An Archaeology of Medical Perception*. New York: Vintage Books, 1994.

Forster, Jean-Paul. "The Gravesian Poem or Language Ill-Treated." *English Studies: A Journal of English Language and Literature* 60 (1979): 471–83. doi:10.1080/00138387908597987.

Freud, Sigmund. *On Aphasia: A Critical Study*. New York: International Universities Press, Inc., 1953.

—. "Psychopathology of Everyday Life." In *The Basic Writings of Sigmund Freud*. Edited and translated by Dr A. A. Brill. New York: The Modern Library, 1995.

—. *The Freud Reader*. Edited by Peter Gay. New York: Norton, 1989.

Friend, Cliff and Billy Rose. "You Tell her I Stutter." Performed by the Happiness Boys, 1923.

Furst, Lilian R. "A Question of Choice in the Naturalistic Novel: Zola's *Thérèse Raquin* and Dreiser's *An American Tragedy*." In Proceedings of the Comparative Literature Symposium. Lubbock: The Texas Tech Press, 1972, 39–53.

Fussell, Paul. *The Great War and Modern Memory*. Oxford and New York: Oxford University Press, 1977.

Gardner, Howard. *The Shattered Mind: The Person After Brain Damage*. New York: Vintage, 1974.

Gay, Carol. "The Fettered Tongue: A Study of the Speech Defect of Cotton Mather." *American Literature* 46, 4 (January 1975): 451–64. http://www.jstor.org.

Genette, Gérard. *Figures II*. Paris: Éditions du Seuil, 1969.

Glauber, I. Peter. "Psychoanalytic Concepts of the Stutter." *The Nervous Child* 2, 2 (1943): 172–80.

Goodglass, Harold and Sheila Blumstein, eds. *Psycholinguistics and Aphasia*. Baltimore: Johns Hopkins University Press, 1973.

"Goody Groaner: The Celebrated Stammering Glee." Eighteenth century ballad.

Graves, Robert. *Collected Poems*. London: Cassell Publishers Limited, 1975.

—. *Collected Poems: Volume 1*. Manchester: Carcanet Press, 1999.

—. *Claudius the God and his wife Messalina*. New York: Vintage International, 1989.

—. *Good-bye to All That*. New York: Anchor Books, 1998.

—. *I, Claudius*. New York: Vintage International, 1989.

Greene, Graham. *Our Man in Havana*. London: Vintage Books, 2006.

Greven, David. "Flesh in the Word: *Billy Budd, Sailor*, Compulsory Homosociality, and the Uses of Queer Desire." *Genders* 37 (2003). http://www.genders.org/g37/g37_greven.html.

Hale, Dorothy. "As I Lay Dying's Heterogeneous Discourse." *NOVEL: A Forum on Fiction* 23, 1 (Autumn 1989): 5–23. http://www.jstor.org.

Hale, Sheila. *The Man Who Lost His Language*. New York: Penguin Books, 2003.

Halvorson, Jerry. *Abandoned: Now Stutter My Orphan*. Hager City, Wisconsin: Halvorson Farms of Wisconsin, Inc., 1999.

Harrison, Casey. "Redemptive Violence and stuttering across the Atlantic: The Who's 'My Generation' and Herman Melville's *Billy Budd* in historical perspective." *Atlantic Studies* 8, 1 (2011): 49–68. doi:10.1080/14788810.2011.539787.

Head, Henry, *Aphasia and Kindred Disorders of Speech: In Two Volumes*. New York; London: Hafner Publishing Company, 1963.

Hecht, Jennifer Michael. *The End of the Soul: Scientific Modernity, Atheism, and Anthropology in France*. New York: Columbia University Press, 2003.

Heller-Roazen, Daniel. *Echolalias*. New York: Zone Books, 2005.

Henry, Anne. " 'Explorations in Dot-and-Dashland': George Meredith's Aphasia." *Nineteenth Century Literature* 61, 3 (2006): 311–42. http://www.jstor.org.

Hipp, Daniel. *The Poetry of Shell Shock: Wartime Trauma and Healing in Wilfred Owen, Ivor Gurney and Siegfried Sassoon*. Jefferson, North Carolina; London: McFarland & Company, Inc., 2005.

Hjelmblink, Finn, Cecilia Bernsten, Hakan Uvhagen, Stefan Kunkel and Inger Holmstrom. "Understanding the meaning of rehabilitation to an aphasic patient through phenomenological analysis – a case study." *International Journal of Qualitative Studies on Health and Wellbeing* 2 (2007): 93–100. doi:10.1080/17482620701296358.

Hockett, Charles F. *A Course in Modern Linguistics.* New York: The Macmillan Company, 1958.

Hoffman, Michael J. "Gertrude Stein in the Psychology Laboratory." *American Quarterly* 17, 1 (Spring 1965): 127–32. http://www.jstor.org.

Horgan, A. D. *Johnson on Language: An Introduction.* New York: St. Martin's Press, 1994.

Hughlings Jackson, John. *Selected Writings: Volume One on Epilepsy and Epileptiform Convulsions.* New York: Basic Books, Inc., 1958.

Hurt, James. "Arthur Kopit's *Wings* and the Languages of the Theater." *American Drama* 8 (1998): 75–94.

Itard, Jean M. G. "Mémoire sur Quelques Fonctions Involontaires des Appareils de la Locomotion, de la Préhension et de la Voix." *Archives Générales de Médecine* 8 (1825): 385–407.

Jacyna, L. S. *Lost Words: Narratives of Language and the Brain: 1825-1926.* Princeton, NJ: Princeton University Press, 2000.

—. *Medicine and Modernism: A Biography of Sir Henry Head.* London: Pickering and Chatto, 2008.

Jakobson, Roman. *Child Language, Aphasia, and Phonological Universals.* New York: Mouton de Gruyter, 1968.

—. *Selected Writings.* New York: Mouton de Gruyter, 1982.

Jakobson, Roman and Morris Halle. *Fundamentals of Language.* New York: Mouton de Gruyter, 2002.

James, William. *The Principles of Psychology: Authorized Edition in Two Volumes.* New York: Dover Publications, Inc., 1950.

Johnson, Jeffrey K. "The Visualisation of the Twisted Tongue: Portrayals of Stuttering in Film, Television, and Comic Books." *The Journal of Popular Culture* 41, 2 (2008): 245–61. doi:10.1111/j.1540-5931.2008.00501.x.

Johnson, Samuel. *A Dictionary of the English Language: An Anthology.* London: Penguin Books, 2005.

—. The *Letters of Samuel Johnson*, five vols, edited by Bruce Redford. The Hyde Edition. New Jersey: Princeton University, 1992.

Jones, David. *In Parenthesis.* New York: Penguin Books, 1963.

Jones, Gail. *Sorry.* New York: Europa Editions, 2007.

—. *Sorry.* London: Harvill Secker, 2007.

—. "Sorry-in-the-Sky: Empathetic Unsettlement, Mourning, and the Stolen Generations." In *Imagining: Literature and Culture in the New World*. Edited by Judith Ryan and Chris Wallace-Crabbe. Cambridge, MA: Harvard University Press, 2004, 159–71.

Joyce, James. *Critical Writings*. Edited by Ellsworth Mason and Richard Ellmann. New York: Cornell University Press, 1989.

Karenberg, Axel. "Cerebral Localisation in the Eighteenth Century – An Overview." *Journal of the History of the Neurosciences* 18 (2009): 248–53. doi:10.1080/09647040802026027.

Kesey, Ken. *One Flew Over the Cuckoo's Nest*. New York: Penguin Books, 2002.

Kopt, Arthur. *Wings*. New York: A Mermaid Drama Book, Hill and Wang, A Division of Farrar, Straus and Giroux, 1978.

Kosinski, Jerzy N. *The Painted Bird*. New York: Grove Press, 1976.

Kravitz, Bennett. *Representations of Illness in Literature and Film*. Newcastle: Cambridge Scholars Publishing, 2010.

Krzywkowski, Isabelle. *Le Temps et l'Espace sont morts hier Les années 1910-1920: Poésie et poétique de la première avant-garde*. Paris: Édition L'improviste, 2006.

Kushner, Howard I. *A Cursing Brain?: The Histories of Tourette Syndrome*. Boston: Harvard University Press, 2000.

Larousse, Pierre. *Grand dictionnaire universel du XIXe siècle*. Paris: Larousse et Boyer, 1865–90.

LeBrun, Yvan, Jacques Flament, Jean Brihaye and Janine-Hasquin Deleval. "L'aphasie de Charles Baudelaire." *Revue Neurologique* 125, 4 (October 1971): 310–6.

Leese, Peter. *Shell Shock: Traumatic Neurosis and the British Soldiers of the First World War*. Hampshire and New York: Palgrave Macmillan, 2002.

Legrenzi, Paolo, Carlo Umilta and Frances Anderson. *On the Limits of Brain Science*. Oxford; New York: Oxford University Press, 2011.

Lehrer, Jonah. *Proust Was a Neuroscientist*. New York: Mariner Books, 2008.

Lethem, Jonathan. *Motherless Brooklyn*. New York: First Vintage Contemporaries, 2000.

Lévy, Bernard-Henri. *Les derniers jours de Charles Baudelaire*. Paris: Éditions Grasset & Fasquelle, 1988.

Lodge, David. "The Language of Modernist Fiction: Metaphor and Metonymy." In *Modernism 1890-1930*, edited by Malcolm Bradbury and James McFarlane. New York: Penguin Books, 1976, 481–96.

Lovell, Arthur. *Beauty of Tone in Speech and Song*. London: Simpkin, Marshall, & Co., Ltd., 1904.

Luria, A. R. *The Man with a Shattered World: The History of a Brain Wound*. Cambridge, MA: Harvard University Press, 1987.

Mann, Thomas. *Doctor Faustus: The Life of the German Composer Adrian Leverkühn As Told by a Friend*. New York: Vintage International, 1999.

Marks, Herbert. "On Prophetic Stammering." *Yale Journal of Criticism* 1, 1 (Fall 1987): 1–20. http://www.pao.chadwyck.com.

Martin, Meredith. "Therapeutic Measures: The Hydra and Wilfred Owen at Craiglockhart War Hospital." *Modernism*/Modernity 14, 1 (January 2007): 35–54. http://www.muse.jhu.edu.

Masson, David I. "Wilfred Owen's Free Phonetic Patterns: Their Style and Function." *Journal of Aesthetics and Art Criticism* 13 (1955): 360–9. http://www.jstor.org.

McCann, Sean. *A Pinnacle of Feeling: American Literature and Presidential Government*. Princeton, NJ: Princeton University Press, 2008.

Melville, Herman. *Billy Budd, Sailor (An Inside Narrative)*. Edited by Harrison Hayford and Merton M. Sealts, Jnr. Chicago and London: Chicago University Press, 1962.

Meyer, Steven. *Irresistible Dictation: Gertrude Stein and the Correlations of Writing and Science*. Stanford: Stanford University Press, 2001.

Milton, John. *Paradise Lost*. Harlow: Longman, an imprint of Pearson Education Limited, 1998.

Mishima, Yukio. *Sun and Steel*. Translated by John Bester. Tokyo; New York; London: Kosansha International, 1980.

—. *Temple of the Golden Pavilion*. New York: Everyman's Library, 1994a.

—. *The Temple of the Golden Pavilion*. New York: Vintage International, 1994b.

Mitchell, David. *Black Swan Green*. New York: Random House Trade Paperbacks, 2007.

Mitterand, Henri, ed., Introduction to *Oeuvres completes* by Émile Zola (*Thérèse Raquin* in Vol.1). Paris: Cercle du Livre Précieux, 1960–7.

Mitterand, Henri. "L'Espace du Corps dans le Roman Realiste." In *Au bonheur des mots: Mélanges en l'honneur de Gérald Antoine* edited by Gerald Antoine. Nancy: PU de Nancy, 1984, xxi.

Morris, David B. *Illness and Culture in the Postmodern Age*. Berkeley: University of California Press, 2000.

Moss, C. Scott. *Recovery With Aphasia: The Aftermath of My Stroke*. Chicago: University of Illinois Press, 1972.

Mukherjee, Ankhi. *Aesthetic Hysteria: The Great Neurosis in Victorian Melodrama and Contemporary Fiction (Literary Criticism and Cultural Theory)*. New York: Routledge, 2007.

Murray, T. J. "Dr Samuel Johnson's movement disorder." *British Medical Journal* 1 (June 1979): 1610–4.

Nelson, Brian. Introduction to *Thérèse Raquin* by Émile Zola. Bristol: Bristol Classical Press, 1992, xiii–xxxi.

Norgate, Paul. "Shell-shock and Poetry: Wilfred Owen at Craiglockhart Hospital." *The Journal of the English Association* 36, 154 (Spring 1987): 1–35. doi:10.1093/english/36.154.1.

Nyström, Maria. "Aphasia – An Existential Loneliness: A Study on the Loss of the World of Symbols." *International Journal of Qualitative Studies on Health and Well-being* 1 (2006): 38–49. doi:10.1080/17482620500501883.

"Oh Helen." Performed by Arthur Fields and Chorus. Edison Records, 1919.

O'Hara, Geoffrey. (1917) "K-K-K-Katy: The Sensational Stammering Song Success Sung by Soldiers and Sailors." Performed by Billy Murray, Edison Records, 1918.

Olson, Charles. *Call Me Ishmael*. New York: Reynal and Hitchcock, 1947.

O'neill, Ynez Violé. *Speech and Speech Disorders in Western Thought Before 1600*. London: Greenwood Press, 1980.

Otomo, Rio. "A Manifestation of Modernity: The Split Gaze and the Oedipalised Space of *The Temple of the Golden Pavilion* by Mishima Yukio." *Japanese Studies* 23, 3 (2003): 277–91. doi:10.1080/1037139032000156351.

Otter, Samuel. "Introduction: Melville and Disability." *Leviathan* 8, 1 (2006): 7–16. doi:10.1111/j.1750-1849.2006.00002.x.

Owens, Wilfred. *Collected Letters*. Edited by Harold Owen and John Bell. London: Oxford University Press, 1967.

—. ed., *Hydra*. Edinburgh: Craiglockhart War Hospital, 1 September 1917.

—. *The Collected Poems*. New York: A New Directions Book, Chatto and Windus Ltd., 1963.

Parr, Susie, Sally Byng and Sue Gilpin, with Chris Ireland. *Talking About Aphasia*. Buckingham; Philadelphia: Open University Press, 1997.

Parr, Susie, Judy Duchan and Carole Pound, eds. *Aphasia Inside Out: Reflections on Communication Disability*. Berkshire: Open University Press, 2003.

Parrish, Timothy. "The End of Identity: Philip Roth's *American Pastoral*." *Shofar* 19, 1 (2000): 84–99. doi:10.1353/sho.2000.0046.

Pearce, J. M. S. "Doctor Samuel Johnson: 'the Great Convulsionary' a victim of Gilles de la Tourette's Syndrome." *Journal of the Royal Society of Medicine* 87 (July 1994): 396–9. http://www.ncbi.nlm.nih.gov.

Perrotta, Tom. *Election*. New York: Berkley Books, 1998.

Plunka, Gene A. "Staging Aphasia: Jean-Claude Van Itallie's *The Traveller*." *Journal of Dramatic Theory and Criticism* (Fall 1999): 3–16. https://www.journals.ku.edu.

Poeppel, David, and David Embick. "Defining the Relation between Linguistics and Neuroscience." In *Twenty-first century psycho-linguistics: four cornerstones*, edited by A. Cutler. New Jersey: Lawrence Erlbaum Associates, 2005, 103–20.

Pollack, David. "Action as Fitting Match to Knowledge: Language and Symbol in Mishima's *Kinkakuji*." *Monumenta Nipponica* 40, 4, (1985): 387–98. http://www.jstor.org.

Proust, Adrien. *De L'Aphasie*. Paris: Librarie de la Faculté de Médicine, Place de l'Ecole-de-Médicine, 1872.

Proust, Marcel. *A la recherche du temps perdu*, 4 vols. Paris: Bibliothèque de la Pléiade, 1988.

—. *Contre Sainte-Beuve*. Paris: Bibliothèque de la Pléiade, 1971.

—. *Correspondance générale*. Paris: Plon, 1970–73.

—. *Essais et articles, presentation de Thierry Laget*. Paris: Éditions Gallimard, 1994.

—. *Les Plaisirs et les Jours* suivi de *L'indifférent*. Edited by Thierry Laget. Paris: Éditions Gallimard, 1993.

—. *Remembrance of Things Past*, 3 vols. New York: Vintage Books, 1982.

Ribot, Théodule. *Les Maladies de la Volonté*. 14th ed. Paris: Félix Alcan, 1883.

Ritchie, Douglas. *Stroke: A Diary of Recovery*. London: Faber and Faber, 1960.

Rivers, W. H. R. "The Repression of War Experience." *Lancet* (2 February 1918): 173–7. http://www.ncbi.nlm.nih.gov.

Rose, F. Clifford, ed., *Neurology of the Arts: Painting Music Literature*. London: Imperial College Press, 2004.

Roth, Philip. *American Pastoral*. New York: Vintage Press, 1998.

Rothfield, Lawrence. *Vital Signs: Medical Realism in Nineteenth-Century Fiction*. Princeton, NJ: Princeton University Press, 1992.

Rothwell, Andrew. Introduction to *Thérèse Raquin* by Émile Zola. Oxford: Oxford University Press World's Classics, 1992.

Sacks, Oliver. *An Anthropologist on Mars*. New York: Vintage, 1996.

—. *Awakenings*. New York: Vintage Books, 1999.

—. *The Man Who Mistook His Wife for a Hat and Other Clinical Tales*. New York: Touchstone, 1998.

—. "Tourette's syndrome and creativity: Exploiting the ticcy witticisms and witty ticcicisms." *BMJ* 305 (December 1992): 15–16. doi:10.1136/bmj.305.6868.1515.

Salisbury, Laura and Andrew Shail, eds. *Neurology and Modernity: A Cultural History of Nervous Systems, 1800–1950*. New York: Palgrave Macmillan, 2010.

Sassoon, Siegfried. *Collected Poems 1908–1956*. London: Faber and Faber, 1984.

—. *Memoirs of an Infantry Officer*. New York: Simon Publications, 1930.

Schleifer, Ronald. "The Poetics of Tourette Syndrome: Language, Neurobiology, and Poetry." *New Literary History* 32, 3 (Summer 2001): 563–84. http://www.jstor.org.

Sedgwick, Eve Kosofsky. *Epistemology of the* Closet. Berkeley: University of California Press, 2008.

Senelick, Richard C., Peter W. Rossi, and Karla Dougherty. *Living with Stroke: A Guide for Families: Help and New Hope for All Those Touched by Stroke.* Illinois: Contemporary Books, 1999.

Shaw, George Bernard. *Pygmalion.* New York: Penguin Classics, 2003.

Shell, Marc. *Stutter.* Cambridge, MA: Harvard University Press, 2005.

Shklovksy, Victor. "Art as Technique." In *Russian Formalist Criticism: Four Essays,* edited by Lee T. Lemon and Marion J. Reis. London: University of Nebraska Press, 1965, 3–24.

—. "On Poetry and Trans-Sense Language." *October* 34 (Autumn 1985): 3–24. http://www.jstor.org.

Silkin, Jon, ed., *The Penguin Book of First World War Poetry.* London: Penguin Books, 1996.

Smock, Ann. "Tongue-Tied Blanchot, Melville, des Forêts." *MLN* 114, 5, Comparative Literature Issue (December 1999): 1037–61. http://www.muse.jhu.edu.

Sontag, Susan. *Illness as Metaphor and Aids and its Metaphors.* London: Penguin Modern Classics, 2002.

Sprinker, Michael. "Hermeneutic Hesitation: The Stuttering Text." *Boundary 2* 9, 1 (Autumn 1980): 217–32. http://www.jstor.org.

Stallworthy, Jon. "Owen and Sassoon: The Craiglockhart Episode." *New Review* 1, 4 (1974): 5–17.

Stanley, Sandra Kumamoto. "Mourning the 'Greatest Generation': Myth and History in Philip Roth's *American Pastoral.*" *Twentieth Century Literature* 51, 1 (2005): 1–24. http://www.jstor.org.

Stein, Gertrude. *Selected Writings of Gertrude Stein.* New York: Vintage Books, 1990.

—. *How to Write.* New York: Dover Publications, Inc., 1975.

—. *Lectures in America.* New York: Random House, 1935.

Steiner, George. *After Babel: Aspects of Language and Translation.* Oxford: Oxford University Press, 1992.

Stengel, E. Introduction to *On Aphasia: A Critical Study* by Sigmund Freud. New York: International Universities Press, Inc., 1953.

Stone, Robert. *Outerbridge Reach.* Boston; New York: A Mariner Book, Houghton Mifflin Company, 1998.

St Pierre, Joshua. "The Construction of the Disabled Speaker: Locating Stuttering in Disability Studies." *Canadian Journal of Disability Studies* 1, 3 (August 2012): 1–21. http://www.cjds.uwaterloo.ca.

Strecker, Edward. *Their Mothers' Sons*. Philadelphia: Lippincott, 1946.

Tancock, Leonard. Introduction to *Thérèse Raquin* by Émile Zola. London: Penguin Books, 1962.

The Oxford English Dictionary. Prepared by J. A. Simpson and E. S. C. Weiner. Oxford: Clarendon Press; New York: Oxford University Press, 1989.

Tracy, Donovan. *The Glass Doctor*. New York, Lincoln and Shanghai: iUniverse, Inc., 2008.

Van Hulle, Dirk. "Hesitancy in Joyce's and Beckett's Manuscripts." *Texas Studies in Literature and Language* 51, 1 (Spring 2009): 17–27. http://www.utexas.metapress.com.

Van Itallie, Jean-Claude. "The Traveler." In *America Hurrah and Other Plays*. New York: Grove Press, 2001.

Warren, Robert Penn. *All the King's Men*. New York: Harcourt Books, 1974.

Waxler, Robert P. "The Mixed Heritage of the Chief: Revisiting the Problem of Manhood in *One Flew Over the Cuckoo's Nest*." *Journal of Popular Culture* 29, 3 (Winter 1995): 225–35. doi:10.1111/j.0022-3840.1995.00225.x.

Wernicke, Carl. *Wernicke's Works on Aphasia: A Sourcebook and Review*. Edited by Gertrude H. Eggert. The Hague: Mouton Publishers, 1977.

Wenke, John. "Melville's Indirection: *Billy Budd,* the Genetic Text, and the Deadly Space Between." In *New Essays on Billy Budd*, edited by Donald Yanella. Cambridge: Cambridge University Press, 2002.

West, Robert W. and Merle Ansberry. *The Rehabilitation of Speech*. New York, Evanston and London: Harper and Row, 1968.

Whitaker, Haigannosh and Whitaker, Harry A., eds. *Studies in Neurolinguistics, Volume 2*. New York: Academic Press, 1976.

Wiltshire, John. *Samuel Johnson in the Medical World: The Doctor and the Patient*. Cambridge: Cambridge University Press, 1991.

Woolf, Virginia. *Mrs. Dalloway*. San Diego, New York and London: A Harvest Book, Harcourt Inc., 1981.

Wordsworth and Coleridge. *Lyrical Ballads* (1798). Oxford and New York: Oxford University Press, 1969.

Wulf, Helen Harlan. *Aphasia, My World Alone*. Detroit: Wayne State University Press, 1979.

Wunberg, Gotthart. "Hermetik – Anigmatik – Aphasie: Zur Lyrik der Moderne." In *Poetik and Geschichte*. Berlin; New York: Walter de Gruyter, 1989, 241–9.

Wylie, Philip. *Generation of Vipers*. Champaign and London: Dalkey Archive Press, 2007.

Yairi, Ehud, Nicoline Ambrose, and Nancy Cox. "Genetics of Stuttering: A Critical Review." *Journal of Speech and Hearing Research* 39 (1996): 771–84. http://www.jslhr.asha.org/cgi/content/abstract/39/4/771.

Yankowitz, Susan. *Night Sky*. London, New York; Toronto: Samuel French, Inc., 1997.

Zaidel, Dahlia W. *Neuropsychology of Art: Neurological, Cognitive and Evolutionary Perspectives*. New York: Psychology Press, 2005.

Zola, Émile. *Germinal*. London: Penguin Books, 2004.

—. *La faute de l'Abbé Mouret*. New York: Mondial, 2005.

—. *La Terre*. Paris: Cercle du live précieux, 1969.

—. *The Belly of Paris*. New York: Oxford University Press, 2009.

—. *The Débacle*. London: Penguin Classics, 1973.

—. *The Earth*. London: Elek, 1967.

—. *The Experimental Novel: And Other Essays*. New York: Cornell University Library, 2009.

—. *Thérèse Raquin*. Paris: Garnier-Flammarion, 1970.

—. *Thérèse Raquin*. Paris: Fasquelle, 1971.

—. *Thérèse Raquin*. London: Penguin Books, 1962.

—. *Thérèse Raquin*. London: Penguin Books, 2010.

Index

Lightning Source UK Ltd.
Milton Keynes UK
UKHW020048020419

340325UK00005B/297/P